Table of Contents

ENDOMETRIOSIS

The Enigmatic Disease

By

Stephen L. Corson M.D.

First Edition

Dr. Corson is Clinical Professor of Obstetrics and Gynecology, the University of Pennsylvania School of Medicine, Director of the Philadelphia Fertility Institute and Section Head, Reproductive Endocrinology, at Pennsylvania Hospital, Philadelphia, Pennsylvania.

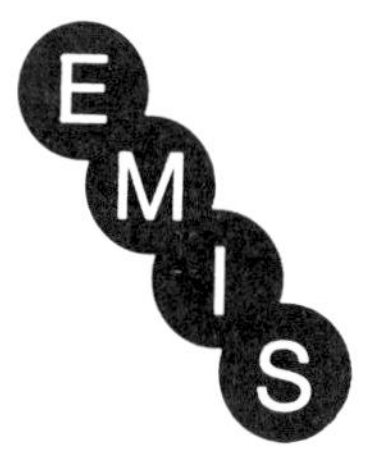

AVAILABLE FROM:

Essential Medical Information Systems, Inc.

P.O. Box 1607

Durant, OK 74702-1607

Essential Medical
Information Systems, Inc.
P.O. Box 1607
Durant, OK 74702-1607

To order, please call:
1-800-225-0694
Fax (405) 924-9414

This book made available through a grant from Syntex Laboratories, Inc. Please see accompanying full prescribing information for Syntex products mentioned in this book.

First Edition
1992

ISBN 0-929240-42-1

Printed in Canada

PREFACE

Endometriosis, the subject of this text, does not easily fit into the usual format of this series of publications. Methods of diagnosis and especially treatment are frequently controversial, and the literature has data from studies which are rarely so well controlled as those, for instance, for managing side effects of oral contraceptive agents.

Nevertheless, without sacrificing accuracy and discussion, an assiduous attempt has been made to present the information in an easily retrievable fashion. References have been chosen from journals which are easily accessed.

I am greatly indebted to Lee Miller for her preparation of the manuscript and to Ray Tschoepe for the artwork.

The laparoscope, more than any other single advance, has had a greater impact first on diagnosis, and then therapy, of endometriosis. With great appreciation I thank Mel Cohen who first put that instrument in my hands some many years ago, and S. Leon Israel who encouraged my early endoscopic efforts.

#1 DEFINITION

1.

Endometriosis is defined as the presence of endometrial glands and stroma outside the endometrial cavity, with the term adenomyosis reserved for lesions within the uterine musculature. Symptoms usually arise from cyclical bleeding into surrounding tissues causing inflammation and scarring, but pain may exist in the absence of hemosiderin deposits. Histologic verification is implied, if not demanded, but in clinical practice diagnosis is made frequently by visual inspection of the peritoneal surfaces via laparoscopy.

These lesions may be active or inactive, pigmented or white, exophytic or invasive, with all morphologies coexisting in the same individual dependent on the maturity of the lesion, site, and previous therapy.

Although usually a benign rather than a malignant process, biopsy-proven endometriosis has been documented in the central nervous system, pulmonary parenchyma and at cutaneous sites.

Aberrant tissue does not always respond in the same fashion as normal endometrium with respect to the usual hormonal changes occurring through the menstrual cycle, nor does it behave in a predictable fashion to therapeutic hormonal manipulation.

Adding to the confusion has been the finding that estrogen receptors have been identified in a minority of endometriotic samples measured [1] in spite of the fact that clinically there seems to be a direct correlation between serum estrogen levels and activity of endometriosis. Progesterone receptors are more commonly found, but some lesions contain neither.

Another possible answer for discordancy between normal endometrium and endometriotic tissue and apparent failure of drug therapy in some cases is that endometriotic lesions often lack critical enzyme systems such as estradiol 17B-hydroxysteroid dehydrogenase[2].

2.

#2 MORPHOLOGY

The diagnosis of endometriosis made by gross morphologic appearance is frequently difficult. First, lesions may change appearance according to the menstrual cycle and previous or current hormonal therapy. Laparoscopically, the operator is dependent on a system which has excellent optics, illumination, and resolution. Abdominal structures must be mobilized and examined on all surfaces. Most important is a commitment to biopsy freely any suspicious areas. Lesions may be pigmented or colorless.

An interesting study was done by Dizerega, et al[3] in castrated monkeys. Experimental endometriosis was created and the animals were subjected to hormonal manipulation. In the absence of continued estrogenic or progestational support, lesions became atrophic. In animals given estrogen, progesterone, or both, lesions were microscopically active.

Vasquez, et al[4] described the morphologic appearance of endometriosis both with light and scanning electromicroscopy (SEM):

- Intraperitoneal polyps with no glandular openings but with deep endometrial glands and stroma.

- Intraperitoneal foci with surface epithelium, glands and stroma.

- Retroperitoneal small lesions with few glands and minimal stroma.

- Mitotic activity as an index of proliferation or secretory activity was not correlated with the endometrial biopsy.

Jansen and Russell[5] called attention to the non-pigmented lesion of endometriosis and defined the continuum between these early implants and the pigmented variety which occur after repeated episodes of growth and regression, bleeding and absorption. Clinically, these early lesions, although less impressive than pigmented ones when viewed laparoscopically, are just as important in producing pain and infertility. Most commonly, histologic verification was seen with:

- peritoneal white opacified lesions (especially when puckering was noted)

- red "flame" lesions which look like endometrium

Lesser degrees of correlation were seen with:

- subovarian adhesions

- yellow-brown patches (tobacco-staining)

- circular peritoneal defects

Some of the patients were followed and relaparoscoped with findings that progression to pigmented lesions occurred in some women.

Chatman and Zbella[6] noted the association between pelvic peritoneal defects and endometriosis (79% positive biopsy diagnoses).

Stripling, et al[7] called attention to pelvic lesions that might be confused with endometriosis, such as ectopic pregnancy, carbon deposits from previous laser or electrosurgical procedures, or retained suture. In another publication, Stripling, et al[8] also reviewed the subject of the subtle appearance of endometriosis.

Martin et al[9] made the important point that endometriotic implants on peritoneal structures and bowel wall were greater than 5mm deep in 25% of patients in whom the depth of the lesion was measured prior to excisional biopsy.

The group from Brussels, headed by Donnez[10] reported a series in which biopsy in 86 women with a visual laparoscopic diagnosis of endometriosis was confirmatory in 93%. But in women not thought to have endometriosis at laparoscopy, biopsy of normal appearing uterosacral ligaments was positive for endometriosis in 6%.

Ovarian endometriomas probably start as surface lesions. The process becomes invasive rather than exophytic with the result that the lesion internalizes with compression of normal ovarian stroma beneath it. Normal tissue then, becomes compressed against the ovarian surface as the cyst enlarges. Various operative techniques have been designed to preserve as much normal ovarian parenchyma as possible and will be discussed in a later section. When tissue response to inflammation is severe, surgical planes are lost and organs become firmly adherent to each other. Masses composed of ovary, tube, omentum and mesocolon are especially common on the left, while ileocecal involvement is frequently seen on the right.

#3 ETIOLOGIES

Samson in 1927[11] advanced the theory of retrograde menstruation with subsequent implantation and growth of viable endometrium on pelvic structures as the etiology of endometriosis. This explanation was supported by clinical findings that lesions tended to be clustered around structures in close proximity to the distal ends of the fallopian tubes with the most dependent portions of the pelvis increasingly involved - ovaries, uterosacral ligaments and posterior cul-de-sac.

Novak[12] carried the concept farther and popularized Meyer's thesis of metaplasia of the mesothelial lining of the peritoneal cavity. This raised the possibility that endometriosis could arise as the result of non-specific irritative stimuli.

Halban[13] proposed that extraperitoneal endometriosis could result from migration of endometrial cells via lymphatic spread. This also answered the apparent enigma of endometriosis arising, or at least becoming clinically manifest, after tubal ligation.[14,15]

Samson[16] described a hematogenous route of spread as another.mechanism for extraperitoneal endometriosis.

Since laparoscopy during menses demonstrates retrograde menstruation into the peritoneal cavity in up to 90% of women[17], the question still remains as to why virtually all women don't develop endometriosis. Ridley[18] demonstrated that endometrial cells found in the regurgitated menstrual effluent from the tube were viable in culture. Genetic predisposition and immunologic failure are only two of the proposed answers to this conundrum.

Epidemiologic studies by Cramer[19] suggest that the total bulk of endometrial cells cast into the peritoneal cavity may be a factor. Women with a greater number of menstrual days (a factor of days of flow and cycle interval) had twice the risk of developing endometriosis as controls. There are also data which suggest that an earlier age of menarche as well as relative menorrhagia serve as contributing factors.

Actually, an apparent increase in endometriosis prevalence may result from more accurate diagnosis, but also may be a consequence of delayed child bearing in combination with methods of contraception other than those which suppress ovulation. Until very recently in human history women in the reproductive age group were either breastfeeding or pregnant, but not ovulating in either case. Women may not be bioengineered to deal with long intervals of repeated ovulation. While this line of reasoning is teliologically attractive, little or no data are available for epidemiologic support.

Smoking and regular strenuous exercise are both known to decrease estrogen levels;[20] hence the findings that exercise may protect against endometriosis and prevalance in smokers may be less.

Studies have shown a relatively high association between endometriosis and obstructed menstrual flow, particularly in the presence of congenital Müllerian abnormalities such as uterine didelphus or a rudimentary uterine horn.[21,22] The diethylstilbestrol (DES) syndrome of intrauterine exposure to estrogens in high dose has not been associated with an increase in endometriosis.[23]

Moen[24] found a retroverted uterus in 47% of patients with documented endometriosis but in only 17% of controls. Whether this is a cause or an effect is unknown.

Notes

#4 PREVALENCE AND HEREDITY

Using women seeking tubal ligation as a control group, prevalence rates for endometriosis were found in two studies to range from 2% through 18%.[24,25] When an infertile population is studied, those rates usually range from 5% through 33% [26-30] dependent on the mix of patients seen.

4.

The range for endometriosis prevalence for women admitted because of pelvic pain is 5% through 21%, and is 0% through 7.1% for admissions because of the finding of a pelvic mass.[26-29], [31]

Actual incidence rates are poorly defined, but the study of Houston, et al[32] in Rochester, Minnesota from 1970 to 1979 suggests a figure of 1.6/1000 woman-years.

Little data exists on ethnic differences. Studies would suggest that whites have a higher prevalence than blacks, and asians have a higher risk than whites.[28,27] However, the notion that black women rarely suffer from endometriosis is incorrect.[33]

That the disease process can be severe in adolescents was shown by Goldstein et al[34] and also by Chatman and Ward[33]. In the former study 47% of 140 patients aged 10.5 to 19 years had endometriosis documented at laparoscopy as the sole etiology of severe pelvic pain. Obstructed egress of menstrual blood was found in 12 as a result of congenital uterine anomaly.

Nine of these had associated urologic anomaly. Unfortunately, follow-up demonstrated recurrence of endometriosis in 29% following initial therapy.

Studies by J. L. Simpson and colleagues[35-36] demonstrated a 6.9% prevalence of endometriosis in first degree relatives (sisters, mothers) of probands versus 1% for sisters or mothers of the patient's husband. Since infertility may result from endometriosis, the actual hereditable influence may be underestimated in the study.

Equally important was the finding that endometriosis on a familial basis tended to be at a more advanced stage when diagnosed, and also acted in a more aggressive fashion.

#5 CLINICAL PRESENTATION AND SYMPTOMS

Endometriosis has been described as an enigmatic, baffling disease with protean symptoms. All of these adjectives and many more have been used to express the frustration of doctor and patient alike in diagnosis and treatment of a disorder with variable morphologic presentation, and frequent poor correlation between the apparent extent of pathology with infertility and pain. Infertility will be discussed specifically later in the text; here we shall concentrate primarily on pain and abnormal bleeding as presenting symptoms. Generally speaking, only active endometriosis with metabolic synthesis within the endometrial glands and hemorrhage causing chronic inflammation and scarring is associated with pain. But often following apparently successful therapy, pain persists and laparoscopy demonstrates the presence of adhesions only and scar tissue as a consequence of the initial pathologic process, and sometimes, as an end result of surgical therapy.

Notes

#6 CLINICAL SIGNS

Pelvic pain often is not discretely localized as a consequence of the anatomy of the pelvic nervous system which carries pain fibers. Usually, pain is most marked just before menstrual flow with extension into the first few days of the menses. Many patients with ovarian involvement report periovulatory discomfort which may persist throughout the luteal phase. Conversely, ovarian endometriomas of considerable size may be symptomless.

6.

Dysmenorrhea, often becoming progressively more severe, is a cardinal symptom of endometriosis. Unlike functional dysmenorrhea found primarily in young women, use of oral contraceptive agents in the usual cyclical fashion produces little relief.

Dyspareunia, is common when lesions involve the lower pelvis, especially the posterior cul-de-sac and uterosacral ligaments. Coital pain is most marked in the luteal phase when implants are most active, but may be present at all times because of chronic scarring and local tissue reaction. Deep penetration during coitus may produce excruciating pelvic pain.

Micturition and defecation pain - implants on the bladder wall and on the colon will frequently produce increasing pain as menses nears. Diarrhea or constipation may accompany posterior cul-de-sac, recto-vaginal septum and/or colon implants. Women often have a history of being treated for chronic urinary disorders, but a thorough history will reveal that the urinary tract infection (so called) always seems to have exacerbation early in the menses.

Ovarian Pain is usually minimal from surface lesions. Continuous dull or throbbing pain may be seen with an enlarging endometrioma dependent in large part on the rate of increase and volume.

Sudden onset of severe generalized peritoneal pain with classic rebound tenderness and occasionally shock is highly suggestive of leakage or rupture from an endometrioma into the peritoneal cavity. Such a clinical situation should be regarded as a surgical emergency calling for laparoscopy or laparotomy.

Pain radiating along the sciatic nerve from buttocks to posterior thigh may be lumbosacral musculoskeletal in many patients, but in young women this symptom especially with menstrual worsening, usually signifies the presence of retroperitoneal endometriosis. Laparoscopy cannot visualize these lesions, which occasionally may be palpated vaginally.

Abnormal Bleeding

Any bleeding from a body orifice other than the vagina which has a cyclicity associated with menses should raise the index of suspicion for endometriosis. This includes melena or frank bleeding from either end of the gastrointestinal tract. Epistaxis or hemoptysis may be a symptom of endometriosis of the nasal mucosa or pulmonary parenchyma. Umbilical endometriosis at the tip of a midline scar, usually following a cesarean section, will often present as a sero-sanguinous discharge. Decidua may implant directly as a consequence of mechanical transfer by the surgeon during the operation.

Vaginal/cervical endometriotic lesions may cause bleeding especially post coitally. These must be biopsied since grossly they cannot be differentiated from melanoma.

Disorders of menstrual cyclicity such as anovulation or metrorrhagia are common and not at all specific for endometriosis. Even with extensive ovarian involvement, ovulation and luteal phase function may be normal according to usual indices. Menorrhagia, however, while nonspecific, is common with endometriosis.

The myth that endometriosis is primarily a disease of thin, Caucasian, career women with compulsive personalties is nothing more than an ex cathedra statement unbuttressed by fact.

As with symptoms, clinical signs of endometriosis evident during physical examination may be nil or marked as a function not only of the total mass of diseased tissue, but also on location and tissue reaction to a chronic inflammatory process. This latter factor frequently seems to be exaggerated compared to the actual bulk of endometriosis present. Prior surgery, when performed in the presence of an active inflammatory process, frequently leaves scar tissue and adhesions as a residue regardless of the skill of the surgeon, who usually encounters significant adhesive disease upon insertion of the laparoscope or at the time of laparotomy. This makes subsequent pelvic examinations less than completely satisfactory with respect to assessing the activity of the disease process. Residual or recurrent pain may be adhesional rather than a result of new lesion formation.

Pelvic Induration results from the inflammation associated with cyclical active bleeding and absorption locally of blood and cellular debris. Local levels of prostanoids and associated macrophage activity may be high with associated pain and scarring. Pelvic ligaments become thickened and indurated, giving a "rubbery" feeling to the examiner. With patients who are cooperative during examination, the ovaries can be felt to be relatively fixed to the posterior broad ligament or to the lateral/posterior pelvic wall.

Pelvic pain on examination then becomes understandable because of this continuing process of bleeding and absorption coupled with local tissue reaction. Pressure on the uterus, deep pelvic examination, and putting ligaments on stretch by cervical movement, may all cause extreme pain. With posterior pelvic disease, examination of the rectovaginal septum between the examiner's fingers exerted into the vagina and anus will cause considerable discomfort. A tender area suprapubically between the abdominal hand and the fingers inserted into the vagina usually suggests anterior cul-de-sac and bladder involvement.

Fixed uterine retroversion, particularly without previous surgery is highly indicative of posterior cul-de-sac endometriosis. Attempts to anteflex the uterus cause extreme pain.

Uterosacral beading is a term used to describe the feel of uterosacral ligament implants that are like small shots or "bee-bees". These lesions actually may be below the peritoneal surface, invisible during laparoscopy, and may need to be approached surgically transvaginally. Moving the cervix laterally to put the ligament on stretch causes pain.

Pigmented cervical and/or vaginal lesions must be biopsied to rule out melanoma.

The asymtomatic pelvic mass is a diagnostic challenge, often requiring additional studies. Pelvic examination may not differentiate between broad ligament leiomyoma and ovarian enlargement. Paratubal cysts are frequently confused with ovarian pathology. The ultrasound examination and laparoscopy are both extremely helpful in elucidating the nature of the findings on clinical examination. In our experience with a series of ovarian endometriomas, 6% presented as asymptomatic masses in a group of patients who were not actively pursuing fertility.

Notes

#7 DIAGNOSTIC STUDIES

Ancillary medical technologies can be focused on the diagnostic challenges posed by endometriosis. Laparoscopy remains the key diagnostic (and therapeutic) tool, but other techniques may be helpful.

The **hysterosalpingogram** (HSG) is a relatively low tech procedure, performed on an out-patient basis in radiology departments. It is an integral part of the initial fertility survey.

7.

- **Endometriosis** is suggested by fixation in elevation of the proximal portion of the fallopian tube (Figure 1).
- **Spiculization** of the dye within the myometrium is almost pathognomonic for adenomyosis (Figure 2).
- **Proximal tubal "cloud bursts"** of dye frequently are associated with salpingitis isthmica nodosa, a fibrotic inflammatory condition of the tube sometimes seen in association with endometriosis.
- **Endometriosis within the tube** may show as irregular filling defects within the lumen.

An Ultrasonic pelvic examination may be:

- Helpful to differentiate between laterally placed serosal or broad ligament myomas and ovarian lesions.

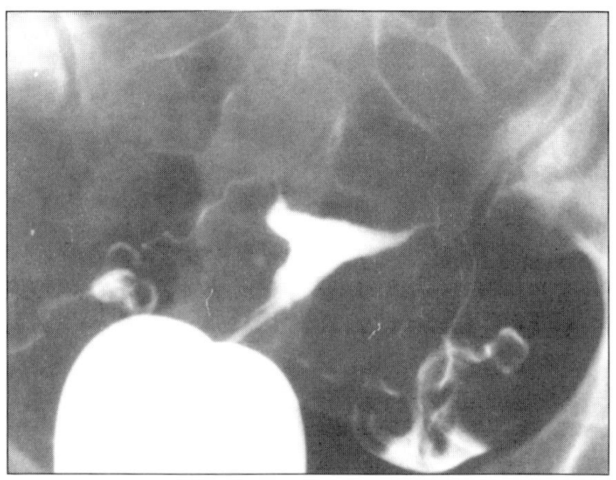

Fig. 1. Elevated and fixed proximal portion of fallopian tube on hysterosalpingography, suggestive of endometriosis.

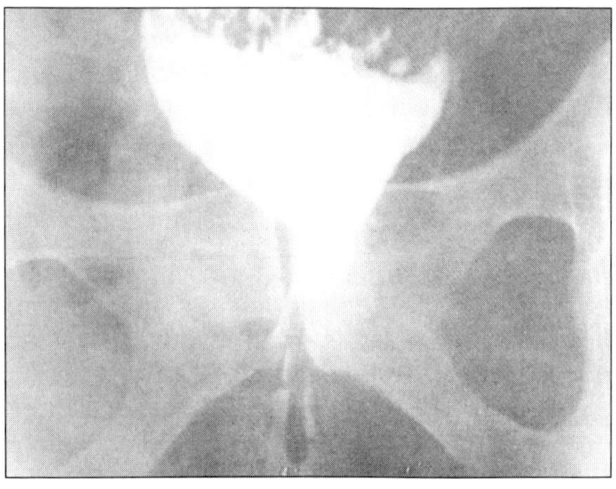

Fig. 2. Entry of dye into the myometrium during hysterosalpingography in a spiculated pattern, pathognomonic for adenomyosis.

- Less accurate is separation of para-ovarian or para- tubal cysts from ovarian cystic lesions.

Ultrasonic demonstration of cystic lesions with papillation and/or excresences, internal or external, denotes the high risk of neoplasia and these lesions should be approached as potentially malignant.

Solid as well as cystic components of the ovarian lesion suggests neoplasia in general, and cystic teratoma quite often. Again, a high index of suspicion should be raised regarding possible malignancy under these circumstances.

High echogenecity within a cystic mass is often found with cystic teratoma.

Ovarian endometriomas usually manifest a "ground glass" appearance on ultrasonography as a consequence of collection of old blood and cellular debris (Fig. 3).

Vaginal ultrasound performed with longer focal length transducers is rapidly replacing the abdominal scan which requires a distended bladder for adequate ovarian visualization. Patients are more comfortable, images are of better resolution, and the study can be performed without waiting for the patient to fill her bladder. In selected patients with laparoscopically documented endometriosis, lesions which reform or appear ***de novo*** can be aspirated with the aid of the vaginal probe in an office setting preparatory to superovulation or in vitro fertilization cycles. Whether the quantity and quality of oocytes retrieved is improved by this maneuver is not yet clear.

Magnetic resonance imaging (MRI) is a diagnostic non-ionizing radiation technique with little new to offer for endometriosis diagnosis except for identification of uterine myoma confused with ovarian lesions and for diagnosis of adenomyosis versus myoma. The images are of excellent quality, but the added information is not cost effective in most cases.

Cystoscopy and/or colonoscopy with appropriate biopsy should be employed when symptoms suggest bladder or colon involvement with endometriosis. Submucosal lesions, not directly luminal, can still cause bleeding and frequently present as focal areas of submucosal puckering. Mucosal lesions are usually pigmented. Proper preoperative assessment will lead to adequate preoperative preparation.

Barium enema as a study is performed when colonoscopy is impossible or technically unsatisfactory. Partial obstruction, presenting as a process mimicking carcinoma of the colon from a collar-like lesion calls for a resection and anastomosis. Apparent fixation and kinking of the bowel during this study also may indicate significant bowel involvement with fibrosis and adhesions.

Other endoscopic procedures may be employed at distant sites as in the head and neck and pulmonary parenchyma.

Hysteroscopy is of some help in identification of adenomyosis, and may also allow for passage of a fiberoptic falloposcope for

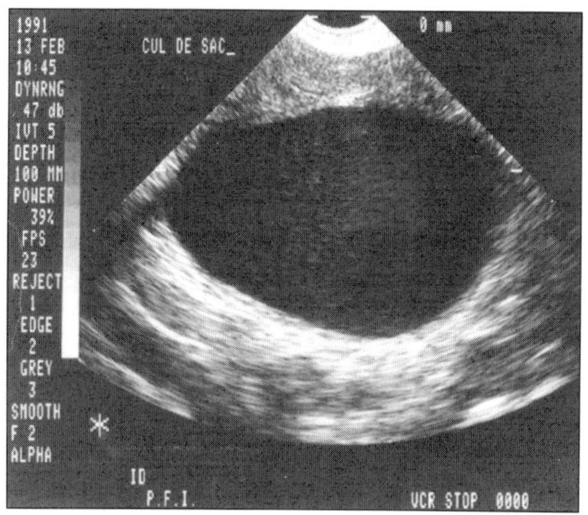

Fig. 3. "Ground glass" ultrasonographic appearance of an ovarian endometrioma.

direct visualization of the fallopian tube lumen in cases where the HSG may have suggested the presence of intraluminal endometriosis.

Laparoscopy is the definitive diagnostic procedure for endometriosis, unless the diagnosis is made secondarily at laparotomy for another indication or because laparotomy has been performed as a consequence of an erroneous diagnosis.

Points to remember are:

- Use general or regional anesthesia rather than local anesthesia to allow for a thorough evaluation of the entire peritoneal cavity.

- An ancillary probe or forceps should be used to completely mobilize the uterus, tubes, and ovaries in order to inspect all of the surfaces.

- Both of the cul-de-sacs and ovarian fossae must be thoroughly examined with adequate lighting, optics, and resolution.

- Lesions may be active or inactive, pigmented or white.

- "Puckering", especially on the ligaments is common with subperitoneal lesions.

- Palpate uterosacral ligaments and the tube with a probe, noting that uterosacral lesions in particular may be quite deeply placed retroperitoneally.

- Biopsy freely, and in particular, any suspicious lesion that is seen.

- Irrigate presumed endometriomas and examine the cyst wall lining internally after an opening has been made.

- Biopsy before application of electrical or laser energy.

- Inspect the appendix for endometriosis; it may be involved in pelvic endometriosis. Likewise, the omentum may be involved with lesions and this should be inspected as well.

Blood studies for diagnosis usually suffer from lack of sensitivity. The sedimentation rate frequently is accelerated, especially when the inflammatory response is brisk. Elevations of sedimentation rate are observed also with any infectious process, neoplasia, regional enteritis, arthritis and other pathologies.

Ca 125 antigen is a glycoprotein of 20 kilodalton molecular weight normally found in Müllerian derivatives, peritoneal, pleural and pericardial cells, and in various fetal tissues. Its serum level is elevated in endometriosis, epithelial carcinomas, pregnancy, pelvic inflammatory disease, adenomyosis and in the presence of uterine myomas. Recent investigations [37-44] have produced the following conclusions.

- Ca 125 antigen can be measured reliably with OC 125 antibody derived from monoclonal mouse cell culture initially immunized to antigen from human papillary serous cyst adenocarcinoma. Estimation can be done as radioimmunoassay or enzyme-linked mmunoassay.

- Most, but not all workers, report that serum levels are higher during menstruation.

- While specificity has been high, usually 0.80 to over 0.90 in most studies, sensitivity has been below 0.20 in most reports.

- Most workers have chosen values of up to 35 U/ml as normal, although Pittaway[38] consistently employes a schema of normal values up to 16 or 20 U/ml.

- In general, there is little or no elevation seen in patients with endometriosis of American Fertility Society Stage I/II.

- Elevations are common in Stages III/IV and can be used to assess long term results of therapy [39,41,43] and prognosis for pregnancy, although there is some disagreement over this in the literature.[40]

- Danazol may have a special immunologic effect in reduction of Ca 125[40] versus medroxyprogesterone acetate therapy, although other progestins as well as GnRH inhibitors have been successful in reducing Ca 125 levels during therapy.[39]

- Follow-up laparoscopic findings of endometriosis activity may[43] or may not[40] correlate with Ca 125 levels.

- Ca 125 antigen determination in evaluation of adnexal cystic formations in young women may be of some preoperative interest in predicting the presence of endometriosis.[38]

#8 DIFFERENTIAL DIAGNOSIS

Usually the patient with endometriosis will present with symptoms of pain of a chronic nature with menstrual accentuation. Coitus may increase the discomfort and if the bladder and/or colon are involved, symptoms referable to these organs frequently will be present. Acute pain of increasing proportions with peritoneal signs points to spontaneous rupture or torsion of an an ovarian endometrioma. In some cases routine pelvic examination will disclose asymptomatic enlargement of adnexal structures. Extraperitoneal endometriosis may present in a variety of bizarre patterns, but cyclical discomfort and bleeding from a body orifice are the most common themes.

Pelvic inflammatory disease (PID) is usually associated with fever, elevated white cell count and diffuse pelvic pain when acute. A cervical discharge with confirmatory culture of a sexually transmitted organism is helpful but not always present. Symptoms tend to be more acute than with endometriosis, but subacute or chronic PID is often confused with endometriosis. The sedimentation rate is of no real help, since it may be elevated with both entities, as is the Ca 125 antigen.

Acute appendicitis is another difficult condition to differentiate from not only endometriosis, but from gastroenteritis and other gastrointestinal disorders. Nausea, constipation, and pain at McBurney's point with fever and leucocytosis are rarely all present. Rectal examination may allow for indirect palpation of the appendiceal tip. As surgeons become more oriented to laparoscopy as a diagnostic modality, the differential diagnosis will be made with increasing accuracy, which should reduce the number of young women operated on for appendicitis who actually have symptomatic endometriosis. Meckel's diverticulitis is less common as a differential diagnosis.

Ovarian cysts of any type may cause pain usually dependent on the rapidity of enlargement and stretching of the ovarian capsule, but torsion, leakage or rupture will cause a constellation of more acute and severe symptoms.

Ectopic pregnancy is another great mimic, and should be suspected when a pregnancy test is positive. Alteration of the menstrual cycle is not always apparent to the patient. Ultrasonography and laparoscopy aid in the diagnosis.

The preceding four acute conditions cause the most diagnostic confusion with endometriosis. Ultrasonography is helpful for ovarian evaluation. Laparoscopy should be performed in cases of PID not responding to adequate antibiotic coverage within 48 hours. Now that surgeons have begun to embrace laparoscopy, at least for cholecystectomy, it is more than likely that they will also employ the laparoscope more often in cases of presumed appendicitis and other acute peritoneal pathologies, especially when symptoms are less than classical, as is often the case when the appendix is retrocecal. Appendectomy, moreover, may be performed more frequently by the laparoscopic route as instrumentation is developed specific for that indication.

Chronic pelvic pain may arise from a variety of sources.

- Adhesional pain from previous infection and/or surgery can be diagnosed and treated (preferably) by laparoscopy.

- Chronic PID, diagnosed laparoscopically, can be treated with long term antibiotics, pain medications, or salpingectomy, if necessary.

- Pelvic congestion syndrome with large pelvic varicosities exacerbates premenstrually. Diagnosis via laparoscopy may be positionally dependent. Ultrasonography is sometimes helpful.

- Intermittent torsion of a cystic ovary will cause pain. More common is combined tubal and ovarian torsion of the distal tubal segment following sterilization procedures.

- Colitis, diverticulitis and regional enteritis can all be confused with endometriosis. Gastrointestinal endoscopy and barium studies of the intestinal tract usually are diagnostic. Rarely, partial obstruction occurs from endometriosis rather than from colon cancer.

It is amazing how many women are treated for chronic urinary tract infection with essentially negative cultures and menstrually related exacerbation of their symptoms. Cystoscopy may demonstrate mucosal or submucosal lesions which can be biopsied to confirm the presence of endometriosis within the wall of the bladder. Pelvic endometriosis affects the ureter more than is realized; intravenous pyelography and laparoscopy are needed to explore this area.

Chronic lumbosacral pain is usually an orthopedic problem, but symptoms can mimick those of endometriosis. Laparoscopy may not completely settle the issue, especially if lesions are retroperitoneal. Often, an emperic trial of drug therapy may be necessary as a diagnostic maneuver.

Chronic dysmenorrhea with or without dyspareunia is a symptom complex not always diagnosed with any modality. These patients may become dependent on analgesics and eventually narcotics. A trial of specific endometriosis drug therapy seems warranted in these circumstances, especially when progestins and antiprostaglandin agents have little or no effect. This is true even when a thorough laparoscopic examination has not proven to be diagnostic.

#9 MALIGNANT TRANSFORMATION

As with all other pathologies which have both benign and malignant components such as serous cysts of the ovary, endometriosis may be malignant. It is not clear whether some malignancies begin as such or progress from benign disease to unchecked neoplasia. With endometriosis there is another possibility; that of neoplasia arising coincidentally in continuity with endometriotic implants.

Sampson[45] in 1925 reported malignancy in endometriosis, with 75% of cases ovarian in origin. His criteria were:

9.

- Coexistence of endometriosis and carcinoma at one site
- Similar histology
- No other primary source
- An additional criterion might be microscopic evidence of continuity between benign and malignant endometrioid epithelium.

Using these criteria, the rate of malignant transformation of endometriosis is probably 1%. A case report by Moll et al[46] documents progression from a typical endometriosis of the ovary to a clear cell adenocarcinoma showing that cell types other than endometrioid can result from the initial lesion.

Heapes et al[47] reviewed the English literature through 1989, and, like Sampson, noted the ovary as the primary source in 79% of 205 cases of neoplasia arising in endometriosis.

Cell types were endometrioid adenocarcinoma (69%), clear-cell carcinoma (13.5%), sarcoma (11.6%), and rare types (6%).

Tumors tended to be low grade, and primary sites were usually radiosensitive in contradistinction to those resistant to chemotherapeutic agents.

Fourteen patients had a malignant tumor in conjunction with estrogen replacement therapy, but five-year survival in this subgroup was 82%. Some patients received progestin therapy following therapy. Reimnitz et al[48] reviewed the issue of malignancy arising from extragonadal endometriosis in conjunction with estrogen replacement following hysterectomy and oophorectomy, and added two cases to the literature.

#10 CLASSIFICATION

The classification system most used is the revised American Fertility Society version of 1985.[49] The actual classification system and some examples, as originally published, appear on the next two pages (Figure 4, 5). This classification replaced the previous one utilized by the American Fertility Society[50], and the widely used classification system of Acosta et al[51].

No one system, especially when formulated by a committee, will please everyone.

- With the 1985 revised classification, more attention is paid to the total three dimensional volume of the endometriosis.
- Additional weighting is also given to the depth of invasion.
- Ovarian scores are quite different from peritoneal lesions.
- Additional weighting is given for bilateral tubal and/or ovarian dense adhesions.

- Greater emphasis has been placed on obliteration of the cul-de-sac.

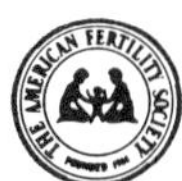

THE AMERICAN FERTILITY SOCIETY
REVISED CLASSIFICATION OF ENDOMETRIOSIS

Patient's Name ________________ Date ________________

Stage I (Minimal) - 1-5
Stage II (Mild) - 6-15
Stage III (Moderate) - 16-40
Stage IV (Severe) - >40
Total ________________

Laparoscopy ________ Laparotomy ________ Photography ________
Recommended Treatment ________________

Prognosis ________________

	ENDOMETRIOSIS	<1cm	1-3cm	>3cm
PERITONEUM	Superficial	1	2	4
	Deep	2	4	6
OVARY	R Superficial	1	2	4
	Deep	4	16	20
	L Superficial	1	2	4
	Deep	4	16	20

POSTERIOR CULDESAC OBLITERATION	Partial	Complete
	4	40

	ADHESIONS	<1/3 Enclosure	1/3-2/3 Enclosure	>2/3 Enclosure
OVARY	R Filmy	1	2	4
	Dense	4	8	16
	L Filmy	1	2	4
	Dense	4	8	16
TUBE	R Filmy	1	2	4
	Dense	4*	8*	16
	L Filmy	1	2	4
	Dense	4*	8*	16

*If the fimbriated end of the fallopian tube is completely enclosed, change the point assignment to 16.

Additional Endometriosis: ________________

Associated Pathology: ________________

To Be Used with Normal Tubes and Ovaries

To Be Used with Abnormal Tubes and/or Ovaries

Fig. 4. From Revised American Fertility Society Classification of Endometriosis:1985. Fertil Steril 43:351, 1985. Reproduced with permission of the publisher, The American Fertility Society.

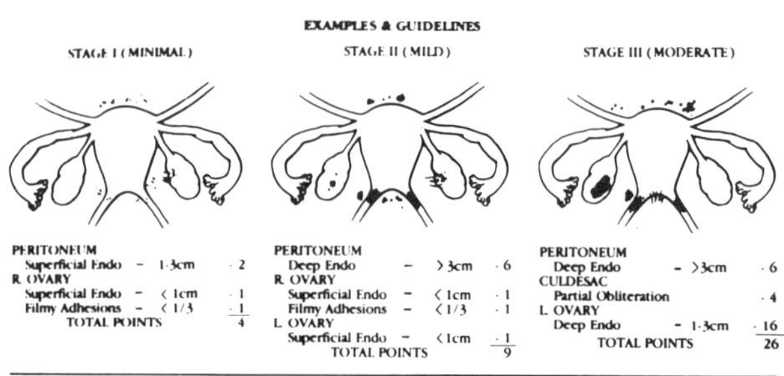

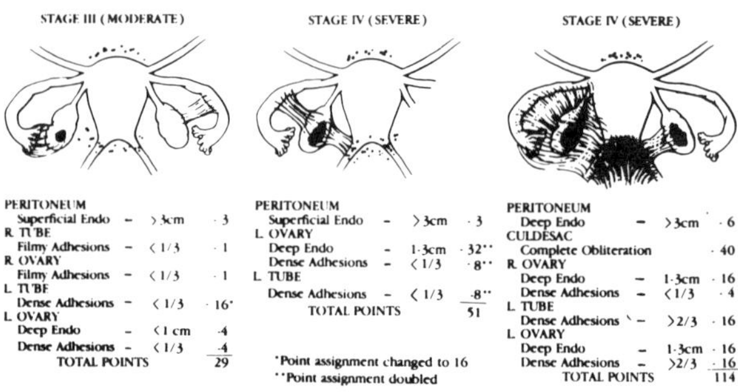

Fig. 5. Examples of Classification System in use. From Revised American Fertility Society Classification of Endometriosis:1985. Fertil Steril 43:351, 1985. Reproduced with permission of the publisher, The American Fertility Society.

Among the criticisms of any classification have been:

- Visual assessment is always subjective, even when video tapes can be scrutinized by different observers.

- It is very difficult to measure the depth of penetration.

- The classification systems are based primarily on anatomic distribution.

- Scoring systems are somewhat arbitrary, particularly with respect to size of endometriomas.

- The morphology of the lesions and the natural history of development is not a factor in assigning a score.
- As with any system, the literature documents investigations of therapies, either drug, surgical, or combination forms, which sometime have a low correlation between success and scores or stages. Whether this is more common in the revised classification as compared with the Acosta version is debatable.

Any system which is utilized should be one which will be both accurate and easy enough to use so that the majority of workers will employ it. It should be a scoring system which has a good prognostic index for pregnancy both with expectant management, and with any of the other active therapeutic modalities. Perhaps the morphology of the lesions and the duration of presence should be factored in as well.

#11 PERITONEAL ANATOMIC DISTRIBUTION

If retrograde menstruation is responsible in large part for initation of endometriosis in those women susceptible to implantation on peritoneal surfaces, then the anatomic location of lesions should show a pattern consistent with that hypothesis. An excellent study of this question was conducted by Jenkins, Olive and Haney[52]. One operator assessed anatomic distribution in 182 consecutive patients laparoscoped for pain and infertility who had lesions of endometriosis. Table 1 and Figure 6 are adapted from that study. The ovary was the most commonly involved site with 100 patients manifesting unilateral or bilateral involvement. Other posterior compartment structures such as the cul-de-sac and uterosacral ligaments were affected frequently. Consistent with the hypothesis, the posterior broad ligament was the site of lesions in 35.2%. Fully 68.1% had posterior compartment endometriosis versus 35.7% for the anterior compartments. Only 10.7% had anterior lesions alone.

Noteworthy was the finding of extensive adhesion formation which usually involved ovary, tube and broad ligament prior to active surgical intervention. Uterine position was evaluated with
11. the finding that 62.1% had anterior uteri, 9.9% had a mid-positional attitude, and 28% had a posterior orientation. Fully 40.7% with anterior uteri had anterior compartment endometriosis.

Results clearly substantiate the interaction between retrograde menstruation and gravity.

TABLE 1
ANATOMIC DISTRIBUTION OF ENDOMETRIOSIS

Location	Implants		Adhesions	
	No. patients	%	No. patients	%
Anterior cul-de-sac	63	34.6	4	2.2
Posterior cul-de-sac	62	34.0	20	11.0
Right ovary	57	31.3	26	14.3
Left ovary	81	44.0	45	24.7
Right anterior broad ligament	2	1.1	2	1.1
Left anterior broad ligament	0	0	3	1.6
Right round ligament	1	.5	2	1.1
Left round ligament	1	.5	2	1.1
Right fallopian tube	3	1.6	20	11.0
Left fallopian tube	8	4.3	28	15.4
Right posterior broad ligament	39	21.4	30	16.5
Left posterior broad ligament	46	25.2	50	27.5
Right uterosacral ligament	28	15.3	5	2.7
Left uterosacral ligament	38	20.8	8	4.4
Uterus	21	11.5	6	3.3
Sigmoid	7	3.8	22	12.1
Right ureter	3	1.6	0	0
Left ureter	2	1.1	3	1.6
Anterior bladder flap	1	.5	1	0.5
Small bowel	1	.5	4	2.2
Anterior abdominal wall	0	0	3	1.6
Omentum	0	0	4	2.2

From Jenkins S, Olive DL, Haney AF: Endometriosis: Pathogenic Implications of this Anatomic Distribution, Obstet Gynecol 67:335, 1986. Reproduced with permission from the American College of Obstetricians and Gynecologists.

Posterior retrodisplacement of the uterus dramatically reduces the anterior cul-de-sac as an anatomic pocket and endometriosis there under those circumstances becomes minimal. Lesions anteriorly were more common in the presence of marked uterine anteflextion. Another factor to be considered is the inherent ability of the tissue to support implantation and growth of endometrial cells. The simple cuboidal epithelium of the peritoneum serves as a better host than stratified epithelium of the cervix and vagina. The ovary seems to be a favored locus, perhaps not only as a consequence of proximity to the tube, but also because of high local concentrations of estrogen and progesterone. Another ingredient may be the monthly trauma at the site of ovulation. Juxtaposition of relatively non-mobile organs accounts for the findings of adhesion formation between ovary and broad ligament.

A separate issue to consider is the relationship between stage of disease and location of pain. A study by Fedele et al[53] noted the following in a group of 160 women with endometriosis.

- 78% had dysmenorrhea
- 39% suffered from pelvic pain
- 32% reported deep dyspareunia
- All three symptoms were found in 17%
- No correlation between pain, presence and/or severity and AFS stage was found
- No correlation existed between symptoms and location of lesions

Lack of correlation with the AFS scoring system may be a consequence of that classification having an orientation leaning more towards fertility evaluation than pain.

Intraperitoneal Organs

Endometriosis has been described in [54]:

- Appendix
- Bowel
- Gallbladder
- Stomach
- Spleen
- Liver

Figures 7-9 show the CAT scan, gross appearance and histologic appearance of endometriosis of the liver.[55] In our practice we have under our care a woman previously unreported who has a history of recurrent pancreatitis flaring during the menses with characteristic enzymatic changes and clinical presentation. She has been on suppressive therapy with gonadotropin releasing hormone agonist (GnRH-a), without recurrence of symptoms. The diagnosis of endometriosis of the pancreas has not been biopsy proven in this case, but rests on solid chemical and clinical evidence.

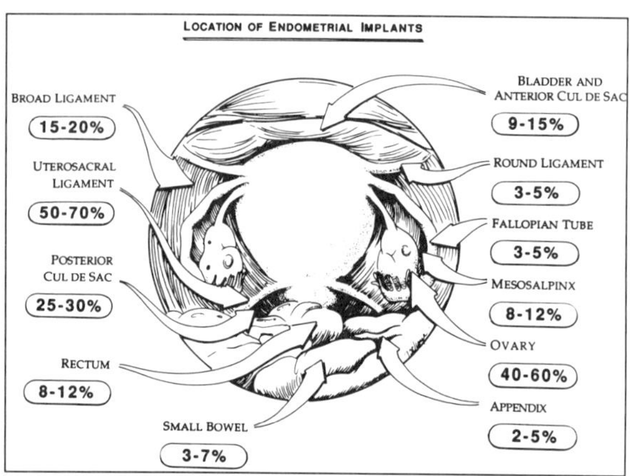

Fig. 6. Location of Endometrial Implants. From Jenkins S, Olive DL, Haney AF: Endometriosis: Pathogenic Implications of this Anatomic Distribution, Obstet Gynecol 67:335, 1986. Reproduced with permission from the American College of Obstetricians and Gynecologists.

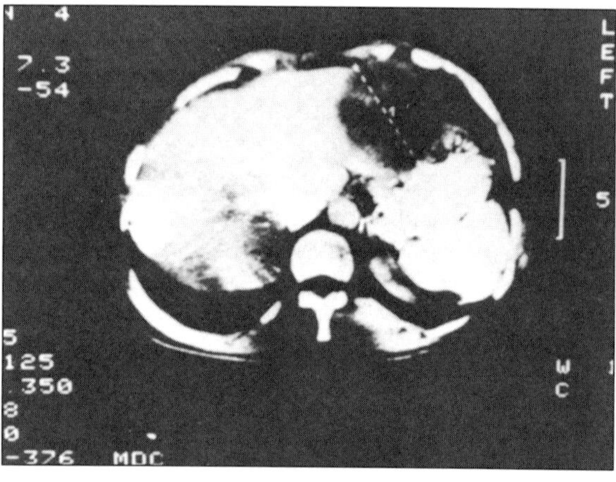

Fig. 7. CAT scan appearance of hepatic endometriosis. From Rovati V, Faleschini E, Vercellini P, Nervetti G, Tagliabue G, Benzi G: Endometrioma of the liver, Am J of Obstet Gynecol 163:1490, 1990. Reprinted with permission from the publisher, Mosby-Year Book Inc.

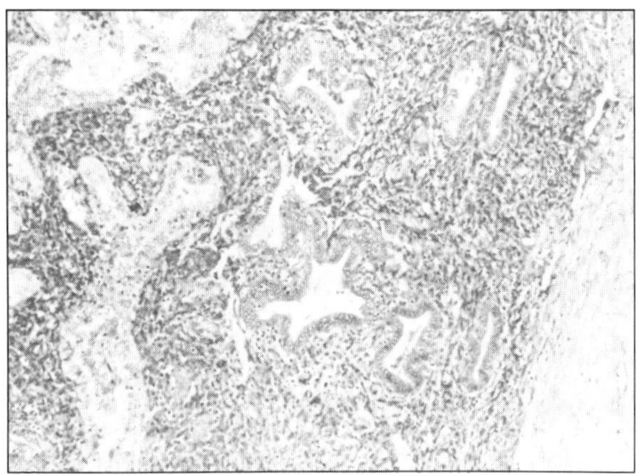

Fig. 8. Histologic appearance of hepatic endometriosis. From Rovati V, Faleschini E, Vercellini P, Nervetti G, Tagliabue G, Benzi G: Endometrioma of the liver, Am J of Obstet Gynecol 163:1490, 1990. Reprinted with permission from the publisher, Mosby-Year Book Inc.

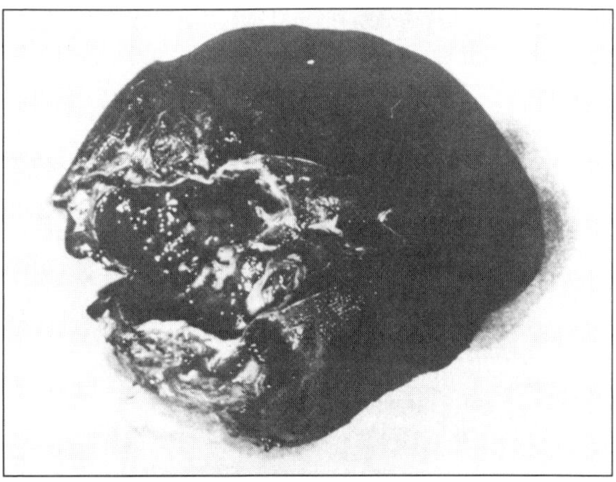

Fig. 9. Gross appearance of hepatic endometriosis. From Rovati V, Faleschini E, Vercellini P, Nervetti G, Tagliabue G, Benzi G: Endometrioma of the liver, Am J of Obstet Gynecol 163:1490, 1990. Reprinted with permission from the publisher, Mosby-Year Book Inc.

Endometriosis of the Small Bowel [56]

- Quite rare
- May cause small bowel obstruction when the ileum is involved
- May mimick a malignant lesion in clinical course and gross appearance at surgery
- Symptoms are not necessarily menstrually related and include (cyclical) diarrhea, lower abdominal cramping, nausea, vomiting, and pain from partial chronic obstruction.

A review of 204 cases in the literature[57] showed that 81% of individual case reports (108) had obstructive phenomena. Pelvic endometriosis was not always a concomitant finding. Obstruction ranged from complete to partial with volvulus and intussusception reported as well. The ileum was involved alone in 71% and in all but one case of 108 with complete data.

Therapy was resection in 81% with immediate or delayed anastomosis. Hysterectomy and castration was performed in 30% as well. Medical therapy was used sparingly, and always postoperatively.

An earlier review in the British literature in 1960[56] found an incidence of 12% intestinal tract involvement in 7,177 cases of endometriosis, with only 7% having small bowel lesions.

Endometriosis of the Colon[58-62]

- More common than small bowel endometriosis
- Crampy abdominal pain is almost universal as a symptom with premenstrual worsening
- Bloody stools are common
- Diarrhea or constipation result as a consequence of irritative response
- Dyschezia is a symptom with menstrual worsening
- Barium enema findings are usually those of kinking and fixation of the sigmoid colon and anterior rectosigmoid
- Strictures indistinguishable from colon cancer may be seen (Figure 10). Filling defects are also common.
- Confusion with diverticulitis is possible.
- Sigmoidoscopy or flexible colonoscopy (better) may demonstrate mucosal lesions that can be biopsied.
- All patients with symptoms suggestive of endometriotic involvement of the large bowel should be screened prior to any surgical procedure and placed on a bowel preparation for possible incision or resection.

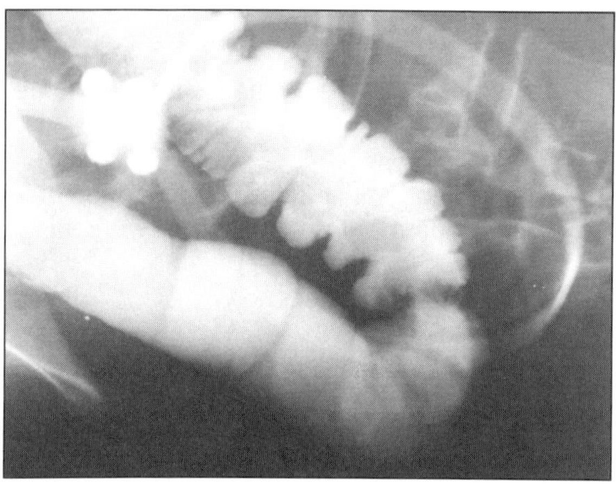

Fig. 10. Barium enema radiographic study of a patient showing colon involvement with endometriosis.

- Hormonal therapy preoperatively usually is not very helpful.
- Rarely, endometriosis of the colon develops as a fistula from a primary ovarian locus.

Weed and Ray[60] reviewed 163 cases of endometriosis of the bowel. Figure 11 and Tables 2 and 3 are reproduced from that study showing the distribution of lesions.

- The sigmoid, rectosigmoid and rectum were involved in decending frequency.
- The appendix was a common site of involvement.
- Resection of implants was the most common procedure performed, but bowel

resection and anastomosis was necessary in 30 cases of large bowel pathology and in 8 ileocecal lesions. There were three temporary colostomies and one permanent colostomy.

- Only one acute obstruction followed surgery.

- Preoperative hormonal therapy was unsuccessful.

- Postoperative estrogen replacement in patients with ovarian ablation was associated with exacerbation of the bowel endometriosis in two patients.

Eliptical longitudinal incisions were made, carried as deeply as necessary, in order to remove lesions with sharp dissection. Fine polyglycolic acid sutures were used.

- In this fashion 73 patients had lesions excised without entry into the mucosa; 13 patients had a mucosal opening.

- Preoperative bowel endoscopy was positive in 42% of 58 patients.

- Barium enema in 29 patients was found to be abnormal in 13.

- Of 153 patients having concomitant gynecologic surgery, 58.8% had extirpation of pelvic reproductive organs.

- Of 54% who could conceive postoperatively, 23 (42.6%) were successful.

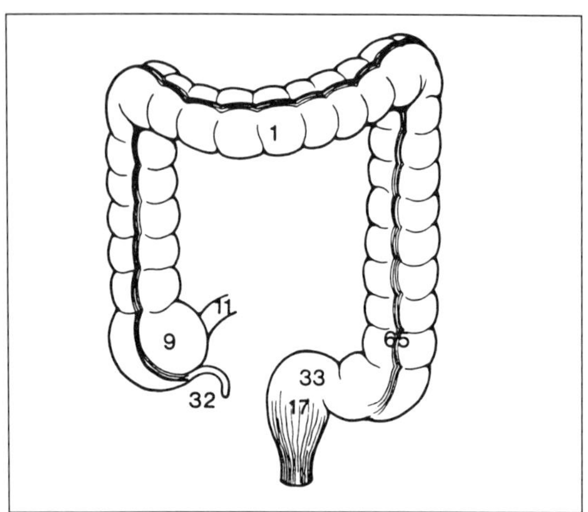

Fig. 11. Anatomic distribution of endometriosis of the bowel. From Weed JC, Ray JE: Endometriosis of the Bowel, Obstet Gynecol 69:727, 1987. Reproduced with permission from the American College of Obstetricians and Gynecologists.

Table 2 shows the presenting symptoms in the 163 women in the study. Other than the one acute obstruction, reoperation was necessary in 33 patients (Table 3) at intervals of up to 13 years.

A group from Baylor[62] reported on 77 consecutive patients with deep colorectal endometriosis treated with full thickness resection. Conservative fertility-promoting procedures were concomitantly performed in 39, and 32 others had oophorectomy with or without hysterectomy. In six patients ovarian ablation had been performed previously. Full bowel resection was performed in 71 instances.

- Postoperative febrile morbidity was 10%.

TABLE 2
PRESENTING SYMPTOMS IN 163 WOMEN WITH ENDOMETRIOSIS OF THE BOWEL

Symptom	N
Endometriosis	
Dysmenorrhea	71
Dyspareunia	39
Unspecified abdominal pain	23
Infertility	39
Suggestive of bowel involvement	
Diarrhea, cyclic	42
Constipation, cyclic	19
Rectal bleeding, cyclic	26
Dyschezia	25
Abdominal distention, cyclic	3
Bowel obstruction, partial	18
Bowel obstruction, complete	1

From Weed JC, Ray JE: Endometriosis of the Bowel, Obstet Gynecol 69:727, 1987. Reproduced with permission from the American College of Obstetricans and Gynecologists.

TABLE 3
REOPERATIONS FOR ENDOMETRIOSIS OF THE BOWEL

Site	Bowel resection (N)	Implant resection (N)	Interval
Colostomy closure	3		60-90 d
Biopsy resection	5		0.2-4 yr
Ablative surgery resection	3*	11†	1-13 yr
Small bowel obstruction	1	6	0.5-4 yr
Conservative surgery–repeat		3¥	2-4 yr
Colectomy		1§	13 yr

* Recurrent endometriosis in one patient.
† Recurrent endometriosis in four patients.
¥ Recurrent endometriosis in three patients.
§ Diverticulosis in one patient.

From Weed JC, Ray JE: Endometriosis of the Bowel, Obstet Gynecol 69:727, 1987. Reproduced with permission from the American College of Obstetricans and Gynecologists.

- Of 33 attempting pregnancy, 13 (39%) were successful.

- No patients had intestinal tract recurrence during a 1-9 year followup.

- Proctosigmoidoscopy preoperatively in 74 cases demonstrated luminal lesions in only two, and mucosal distortion in 15 others caused by submucosal lesions.

- Barium enema studies were abnormal in 18 of 73.

- Relief of symptoms was complete in 49%, satisfactory in 39%, unchanged in 11%, and worse in 1% during the follow-up interval.

- Two patients were reoperated for obstruction in the postoperative period.

The authors emphasize that only resection and anastomosis can fully reverse the effect of fibrosis of the surrounding tissue caused by the implants. Bowel involvement with the advanced stages of endometriosis may be more common than previously thought. Thorough examination preoperatively with ancillary techniques and palpation of the bowel at laparoscopy or laparotomy is necessary to diagnose subtle lesions. Preoperative use of danazol for three months was said to reduce the mass of the implants and to decrease bleeding. Remnant ovarian tissue following hysterectomy with apparent total oophorectomy may be responsible for continued stimulation of the bowel implants. Even complete ovarian removal may not cause regression of bowel endometriosis. The authors agree that postoperative estrogen replacement should not be instituted immediately, and that it can cause exacerbation even years later.

Other Retroperitoneal Endometriosis

Aside from involvement of the rectal wall below the peritoneal line, endometriosis may affect other structures in the pelvis which are retroperitoneal. The ureters are rarely attacked, but obstructive uropathy as an end result is particularly nasty.[63-67] Obstruction may result from external compression and cicatrix formation, or by direct growth on ureteral wall with eventual penetration into the lumen.

- Hydronephrosis ensues, usually with no acute symptoms.

- The kidney on the affected side becomes non-functioning in 25% of cases in spite of therapy.

- Patients may present with hypertension.

- Blood urea nitrogen and creatinine clearance may be normal or abnormal depending on the bilaterality of the process.

- Low back pain or flank pain is rarely severe enough to cause attention to the urinary tract.

- Intravenous pyleography (IVP) demonstrates hydroureter and hydronephrosis with varying degrees of residual renal function.

- Standard therapy is surgical with decompresion if possible, and resection-anastomosis or ureteroneocystostomy, when necessary.

- Hydronephrosis and renal impairment may be permanent because of fibrosis. Hypertension may be only partially relieved following therapy.

- Passage of a ureteral stent catheter via cystoscopy may be a useful temporary decompression procedure and a help at surgery.

- Peritonealization of the ureter after extensive ureteral lysis may prevent continued problems.

Maxon et at [64] prospectively studied 63 patients with endometriosis by high-dose IVP and compared results with a control group (n=84). Only one abnormality was noted in the controls, but 10 (15.9%) of the patients had ureteral abnormalities, usually kinking, extrinsic compression, and/or luminal narrowing within 0.5cm of the ureterovesical junction. In this group of endometriosis patients no actual hydroureter was found. ***The left ureter was involved in all cases;*** the right in only one. Ureteral abnormality was related to higher AFS scores.

A number of publications have examined the role of danazol in the treatment of ureteral abnormality associated with endometriosis.[66-67] Figure 12-13 shows pre- and postoperative retrograde pyelograms which clearly demonstrate left ureteral compromise followed by recovery after surgery plus danazol. In general, about 50% have IVP evidence of resolution after 3-8 months of therapy. Sufficient experience is lacking to evaluate whether drug therapy or hormonal manipulation can relieve ureteral obstruction on a long-term basis. The experience to date would indicate that it can be a helpful preoperative surgical adjunct.

The clinician's suspicions of endometriosis affecting the ureter should be aroused when:

- On pelvic examination there is loss of the posterior cul-de-sac as an anatomic space.
- The process seems to extend laterally to the pelvic wall.
- The patient has chronic urinary symptoms or flank pain.
- The patient has newly acquired progressive hypertension.
- When blood urea nitrogen (BUN) or creatinine clearance is abnormal.

An IVP should be ordered more often as a preoperative diagnostic study.

Endometriomas of the bladder penetrating to the muscularis may cause symptoms that are thought to be cystitis. Patients with endometriosis should be quizzed about cyclically recurring urinary symptoms. Mucosal lesions, which can be biopsied via cystoscopy, may cause menstrually related hematuria.

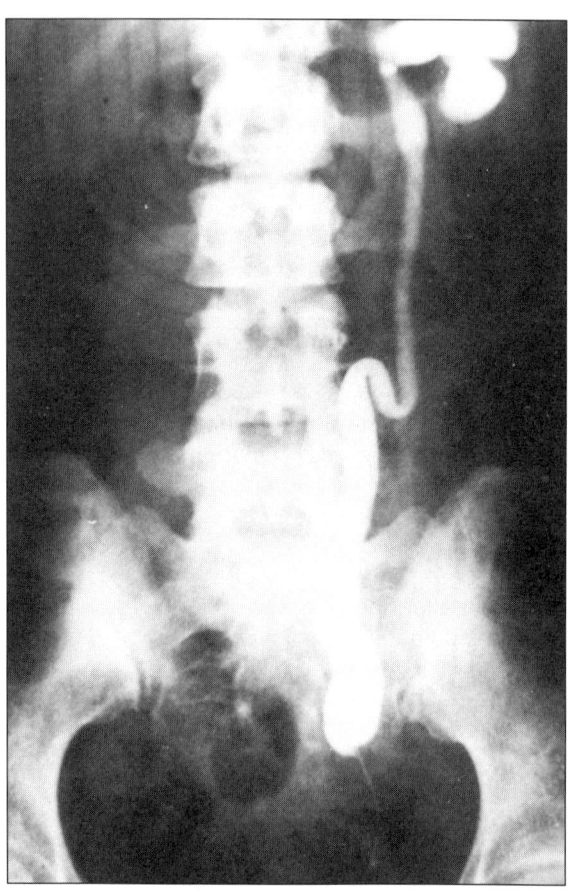

Fig. 12. Pre-operative intravenous pyelogram showing endometriosis-induced ureteral obstruction. From Rivlin ME, Kruegar RP, Wiser WL: Danazol in the management of ureteral obstruction secondary to endometriosis, Fertil Steril 44:274, 1985. Reproduced with permission of the publisher, The American Fertility Society.

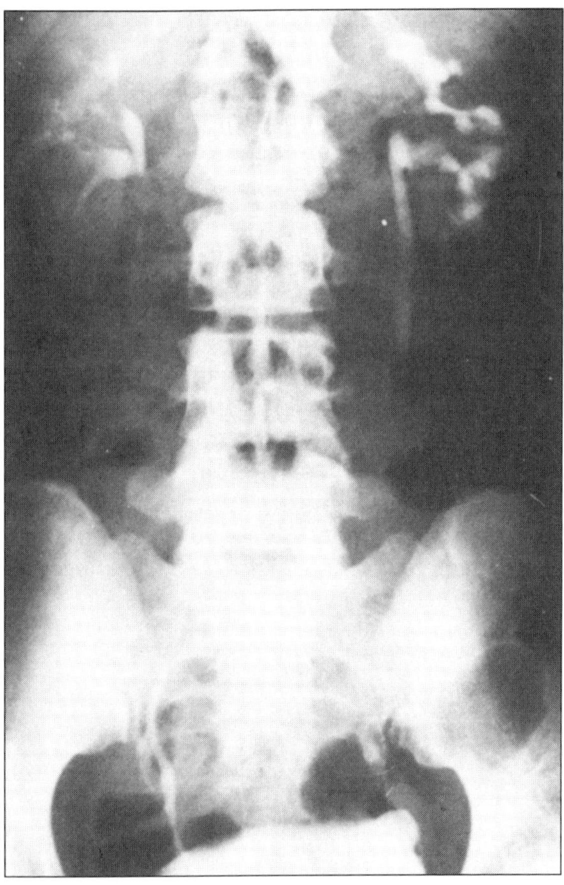

Fig. 13 Post-operative intravenous pyelogram showing clearing of ureteral obstruction. From Rivlin ME, Kruegar RP, Wiser WL: Danazol in the management of ureteral obstruction secondary to endometriosis, Fertil Steril 44:274, 1985. Reproduced with permission of the publisher, The American Fertility Society.

LARGE NERVE INVOLVEMENT

Case reports of deep uterosacral ligament endometriosis causing compression of the sciatic nerve[68] reminds us that symptoms thought to be on an orthopedic basis in a young woman, may, in fact, arise from endometriosis. Also obturator nerve involvement may give rise to pain in the inner thigh as well as causing muscular weakness.[69]

In our practice we have such a patient who has biopsy-proven endometriosis of the obturator space. Rather than risk chronic lymphedema from a radical type of groin dissection, we have treated her with great success using depo medroxyprogesterone for three years, given as 200mg at 90 day intervals.

Notes

#12 EXTRA ABDOMINAL, EXTRA PELVIC ENDOMETRIOSIS

Pulmonary Endometriosis

Foster et al[70] studied pulmonary endometriosis and concluded that both pleura and parenchyma could be involved. Documentation was provided by thoracotomy, chest x-ray, biopsy or catamenial pneumothorax in 65 cases culled from the literature or from observation.

- Patients with pleural disease had symptoms of pain and dyspnea with a *right pneumothorax or pleural effusion in 93%.*

- The mechanism of spread was similar to involvement of the right diaphragm with cases of metastatic ovarian cancer, i.e. cellular migration in the peritoneal fluid flow pattern up the right gutter to the diaphragm.

- 47% had pelvic endometriosis diagnosed previously.

- 19% had experienced previous pelvic surgery.

Patients with pleural disease were more likely to have a history of pelvic endometriosis, and the spread could be accounted for by direct transportation through diaphragmatic fenestrations. Conversely, women with parenchymal lesions often had disease without coexisting pelvic endometriosis. These women tended to be parous and to have a previous history for gynecologic surgery for conditions other than endometriosis. The mechanism of transmission for this group was postulated to be a hematogenous one similar to pulmonary embolic phenomena, especially since the lower lobes (the site of greater blood flow) were most frequently involved.

Catamenial pneumothorax must be distinguished from

- Spontaneous, non-cyclical pneumothorax (more common in men).

- Pulmonary tuberculosis

- Bronchiectasis

- Pneumonia

- Goodpasture syndrome

Parenchymal pulmonary endometriosis may present as cyclical hemoptysis alone. Bronchoscopy during the bleeding episode will usually localize the site of involvement, but this is not true in all cases. Danazol therapy[71,72] is often beneficial, but recurrence upon cessation of treatment is common.

Cutaneous Endometriosis

Cutaneous endometriosis was the subject of an excellent report by Steck and Helwig[73].

- The umbilicus was involved in 28 of 82

patients, with 21 of those unassociated with prior surgery.

- 5 lesions in the inguinal region were also unassociated with a previous surgical procedure.

- 42 cases were in the lower abdominal wall.

- In 56 patients there was endometriosis at a site of a surgical scar, with 26 of those being a cesarean section.

Endometriosis in the last group almost certainly was a consequence of inadvertant direct mechanical transportation from decidua during the surgical procedure. Lesions were:

- Firm or hard

- As large as 6 cm

- Usually pigmented and ranged from pink through brown to blue or black.

In addition:

- Local pain was experienced by 44.

- Cyclical bleeding of the lesion was observed in 10 cases.

- Symptoms worsened at the menses in 33.

- In 15 patients having laparotomy 8 had no pelvic endometriosis.

- Cell lesions exhibited both glands and stroma.

- Every stage of the endometrial cycle was seen histologically and frequently more than one stage was seen within a single specimen.

- A decidual reaction was seen in 9 cases, with 8 of those women being pregnant.

- The dermis surrounding the lesion showed inflammation and fibrosis with both old and acute hemorrhage and an infiltrate of lymphocytes, histiocytes, fibroblasts and iron-filled macrophages.

In summary, extrapelvic, or extraperitoneal endometriosis can arise almost anywhere in the body, probably from hematogenous or lymphatic spread or perhaps from celomic metaplasia. Seemingly unrelated symptoms should cause the astute physician to consider endometriosis as a diagnosis, whether pelvic endometriosis is known to be present or not. Biopsy documentation is preferable, but not always possible. Menstrually related exacerbation of symptoms is a good clue, but is not always present. Drug or hormonal therapy might help, but frequently the explants will not completely respond to hormonal manipulation, and surgery becomes necessary. The decision is based on the risk of the procedure and its complications compared with the potential benefit from this form of therapy.

#13 MEDICATIONS FOR PAIN CONTROL

Non specific analgesics play a role in the overall approach to pain associated with endometriosis. Since prostanoids are thought to be central in the inflammatory process leading to pain, antiprostaglandin preparations have proven popular as a first-line agent of choice. Patients seem to do better when medication is initiated at the first signs of discomfort rather than waiting for severe pain to develop.

Most of the clinical studies dealing with prostaglandin synthetase inhibitors were directed towards dysmenorrhea in general, and primary dysmenorrhea, in particular, without a laparoscopic diagnosis. Studies done with indomethacin, a potent non-steroidal antiinflammatory drug (NSAID), documented relief of dysmenorrhea in association with reduction of uterine tone and high amplitude spastic uterine contractions, probably by local reduction of prostaglandin (PG) levels.[74] Studies have documented high levels of prostanoids in endometriotic implants,[75] and therefore a beneficial effort of NSAID agent is to be expected.

Nevertheless, while early studies documented the advantage of agents such as ibuprofen over aspirin and/or placebo for control of dysmenorrhea,[76] studies specific for endometriosis-induced pain were lacking. Both ibuprofen[77] and naproxen sodium[78,79] were found to decrease PG levels in menstrual effluent.

Therefore, the study by Kauppila and Ronnberg [80] was important, because all of the 20 patients had laparoscopic diagnosis of endometriosis, with active treatment, either medical or surgical, withheld prior to and during the double-blind, placebo crossover trial with naproxen sodium (Anaprox-Syntex).

- Substantial pain relief was obtained in 83% of 40 naproxen sodium cycles versus 41% of 39 placebo cycles (p=0.008)

- No therapeutic effect was seen in 7% of naproxen sodium cycles versus 46% of placebo treatments.

- AFS staging did not correlate with therapeutic response. Note, however, that the dosage regimen of Anaprox (q4-6h) was in excess of the recommended levels (q6-8h) and results might have been different with the approved dosage regimen.

Most physicians are reluctant to employ narcotic and/or codeine-based preparations for control of these symptoms. Perhaps we have become overcautious in this area because of increased awareness of the modern day "drug-culture" within our society. So long as close supervision is maintained, judicious use of these preparations over the course of a few days or a week every month has little propensity to induce addiction, and certainly elevates quality of life by allowing the patient to function on a regular daily basis.

Evaluating pharmacologic therapy of endometriosis with respect to subsequent pain relief is difficult because of the inherent variation of the severity of symptoms from month to month, the subjective nature of the data base and the substantial placebo effect noted in all double-blind studies done for pain control. Incidentally, the literature on placebo-controlled studies for endometriosis pain is notably sparse.

Usually hormonal therapy for endometriosis buys time during which symptoms regress and fertility may be augmented without effecting a cure of any permanence. An interesting study from Brussels documented this by studying biopsy specimens following various hormonal therapies[81]. Mitotic index within the lesions was unchanged from control patients regardless of treatment with progestins, antiprogestins, or gonadotropin releasing hormone agonists (GnRH-a) for six months. Explanations for the findings included:

- Fibrosis preventing drug access to the center of the lesion.
- Dedifferentiation and genetic changes in endometriotic cells decreasing responsiveness to hormonal manipulation.
- Low content of steroid receptors in the implants.

PSEUDOPREGNANCY

One of the landmark articles in the history of pharmacologic treatment of endometriosis was the report by Kistner in 1959[82] on 58 women treated with Enovid* (norethynodrel and mestranol, GD Searle Co.). This approach was taken as a consequence of observations suggesting that pregnancy was prophylactic against development of endometriosis and could actually cause regression of established lesions. Mechanisms postulated included:

- Production of anovulation and amenorrhea.
- Decidual change induced within the lesions.
- Eventual decidual necrosis and absorption.

Medication was begun at a 10mg daily dose of the progestin and increased every two weeks to a maximum of 40 or 50mg. There were actually four subsets of patients in this study, but histologic sections confirmed development of a decidual-like reaction and subsequent necrosis. Side effects included nausea, mastodynia, fluid retention and vaginal discharge. Pregnancy rates following therapy were less than with surgery, but it was hoped that this form of therapy might eliminate surgery for many patents. No mention was made of the often observed phenomenon that patients treated in this fashion tend to have increased severity of symptoms initially before improvement is noted.

Other reports followed between 1961 and 1974 utilizing various oral contraceptive estrogen-progestin combination pills[83-86]. Pain relief was usually 80% or more, and side effects were annoying, related to both compounds. The usual protocol started with one tablet daily and increased to three daily in order to control breakthrough bleeding (BTB).

- Pain was worse for the first two or three months.

- Patients experienced side effects such as depression, mastodynia, appetite stimulation, weight gain, edema, bloating, and sometimes worsening of migraine headaches.

- Pre-existing varicosities frequently became worse.

This form of treatment did not become very popular because of poor acceptance by the patient population as a consequence of both estrogenic and progestational side effects. The doses of both were unusually high by today's standards. Few patients are managed by continuous oral contraceptives today, even with the lower doses and more specific, potent, progestins available.

ESTROGENS OR TESTOSTERONE

The use of testosterone and its derivatives alone to treat endometriosis is of historical interest only because of the associated metabolic side effects. Karnaky[87,88] advocated use of stilbestrol alone to deal with endometriosis essentially by stimulatory exhaustion, but this treatment had short-lived popularity.

MEDROXYPROGESTERONE ACETATE* (MPA)

Figure 14 demonstrates the similarity of MPA to native progesterone, but the synthetic version in animal studies proved to be about 30 times as potent. In its oily depot form it can cause amenorrhea for 3-15 months with a single 200mg injection. An early study was reported by Gunning and Moyer[89] in 14 patients with documented endometriosis. Some patients received estrogens to cope with irregular menses; MPA was given as a 100 mgs at two week intervals over 12 to 31 weeks. Patients were followed for 13-62 months and four of eight with infertility conceived, but eight of 14 had surgery during or following MPA administration. (*Depo Provera - The Upjohn Company)

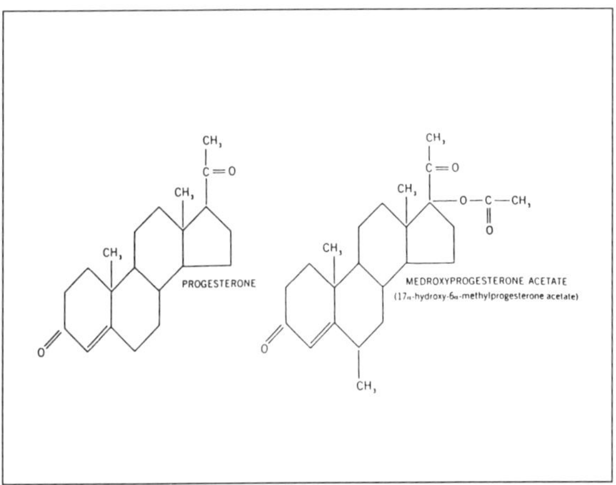

Fig. 14. Chemical structure of progesterone and medroxy-progesterone acetate.

Average weight gain was 4.25 lb; other side-effects were nervouseness, bloating, depression, irritability, and edema. The main problem was that all patients had BTB and menstrual function did not resume until 26 months after the last dose in one patient. Tissue at the time of surgery was noted to be vascular and edematous but with good surgical cleavage planes. Microscopically, the lesions showed an increased pseudodecidual effect.

Thus, this early study documented most of the problems associated with D-MPA therapy.

- Onset of therapeutic effect is slow, with pain relief frequently not apparent for two or three months.

- Storage in the body is prolonged, especially in obese individuals. This limits its usefulness in women wishing to have fertility potential restored promptly after stopping treatment.

- BTB usually is a result of extreme endometrial atrophy in spots, and necrobiosis from decidualization in others.

BTB is rarely a consequence of insufficient dose, and giving greater amounts of MPA at shorter intervals is often counterproductive. Today, the usual dose regimens are 100-200mg at 60-90 day intervals, based on weight and clinical response.

- Treatment for BTB is estrogen alone or estrogen in combination with a progestin such with oral contraceptive preparations for 10-30 days, as needed.

- Progestational side-effects are frequently annoying to the patient and can be ameliorated with concomitant use of diuretics, tranquilizers, hypnotics, etc.

Although structurally similar to native progesterone, and not inherently as androgenic as the 19-nortestosterone compounds, D-MPA causes adverse lipoprotein changes, particularly in the HDL_2 subfraction of cholesterol[90]. This must be considered according to the patient's family history and her pretherapy lipoprotein profile.

Today D-MPA remains a treatment of choice for certain individuals. These tend to be women not desiring fertility who have recurrent disease following short courses of hormonal therapy as well as surgery. If the lipid changes are not great, and BTB is not a problem (it usually ceases after 6-9 months) they can be managed this way over a long period of time with an agent that is less expensive than the GnRH-a agents and which actually controls vasomotor symptoms rather than initiates them. A particularly good candidate for long term therapy is the woman with recurrent endometriosis following hysterectomy with or without ovarian removal. Even in the absence of estrogen replacement, an ovarian remnant or adrenally produced steroids may stimulate lesions left along the vaginal cuff or in the wall of the colon or bladder. D-MPA is very helpful here when given for 12-18 months.

Moghissi and Boyce[91] reported on the use of oral MPA as 30mg daily over a 90 day course in 35 patients. All patients were said to demonstrate improvement or remission, but some had surgery with a follow-up interval of one year. Side-effects were the same as with the parenteral route.

Luciano et al[92] used orally administered MPA, 50mg daily, for four months in 21 women with moderate to severe endometriosis. Patients had laparoscopic pelvic scoring before and after therapy.

- Improvement of symptoms, pelvic nodularity and tenderness was noted in 80%, accompanied by reductions in mean AFS scores from 18.2 to 5.9 (initial classification system).

- Only 71% achieved amenorrhea; 20% had BTB and 10% had persistent cyclical bleeding.

- Estradiol levels were reduced to 46 pg/ml (approximately 140 pmol/l which is not as low a level as that achieved with GnRH-a therapy.

- Histologic change in the endometrium and in the implants was either atrophy or pseudodecidualization.

In spite of this increased dose, amenorrhea was obtained in only 70% of the patients. A prolonged follow-up was not reported, and one can surmise that the typical high rate of recrudescence could be expected. Neither conservative surgery nor pharmacologic treatment permanently alters the mechanism(s) by which endometriosis forms in the pelvis, unless an obstruction to normal menstrual egress has been corrected.

An interesting study was reported by Haney and Weinberg[93], who studied peritoneal fluid volume and total leukocyte content of the fluid before and after therapy of endometriosis with 30mg daily of oral MPA. While reductions in scoring were more modest than reported by others, peritoneal fluid volume dropped appreciably and the total macrophage content dropped dramatically. The authors concluded that retrograde menstruation elicits a sterile peritoneal inflammatory response.

A different story emerged from a pilot study done by Cedars et al[94] in which 20-30mg of MPA was added to a GnRH-a given for endometriosis in eight patients. As expected, this combination reduced or eliminated vasomotor symptoms and loss of bone calcium, but the therapeutic effect of the agonist was blunted as documented by before and after laparoscopic examination. This occurred in the absence of any differences in follicular stimulating hormone (FSH), luteinizing hormone (LH), or estradiol (E_2) levels compared with treatment by agonists alone in a 6 month study. Both AFS scores and a pain index scoring system were unchanged with combination therapy compared with the decrease seen with GnRH-a alone. Such add-back therapy is experimental and not approved for use by either the U.S. FDA or Canadian HPB.

DANAZOL

A more detailed discussion of danazol will be found in the section on infertility in which metabolic changes and side-effects will be treated in greater detail. This section primarily will cover danazol as it relates to control of pain associated with endometriosis. However, since the effect of MPA on lipoproteins[90] was mentioned in this section previously, another study should be included for comparison. Telimaa et al[95] found in a 6 month study that danazol, 600mg daily:

- Decreased HDL cholesterol by 53% versus a 26% reduction seen with 100mg of MPA daily.
- Danazol increased LDL cholesterol by 37%; MPA had no effect.
- Danazol decreased apolipoprotein A-2 levels by 29% versus a 12% negative change for MPA.
- Danazol increased apolipoprotein B levels by 17%; MPA produced no change.

These results indicate that danazol has a much greater potential to produce changes in lipoprotein metabolism thought to be adverse, and which lead to accelerated atherogenesis and possible cardiovascular insult. Long term studies on morbidity and mortality in women having multiple courses of therapy are non-existent.

An early study by Noble and Letchworth[96] compared danazol therapy versus Enovid for endometriosis. Danazol was better tolerated and results for pain relief were better, but a dose of only 400mg daily was used. This study group was rather small, but the results were widely quoted to demonstrate the superiority of danazol over the pseudopregnancy program achieved with the progestins for endometriosis therapy.

A good answer to the question of pain recurrence was provided by a study performed by Greenblatt and Tzingounis[97]. A group of 49 women, 46 of whom had dysmenorrhea associated with endometriosis, received 800mg of danazol for 6 months (a full therapeutic dose and duration).

- Pain recurred in 14 during a 78 month follow-up with a mean of 9 months to recurr-ence.

- Pain was of the same as pre-therapy intensity in 7 and was less in 7.

- Pelvic pain independent of menses was a complaint of 45 of the total group of 49. This pelvic pain recurred in 12, with a mean of only 4.4 months after stopping therapy. The level of pain was unchanged in four and less in eight compared with that before treatment.

This study would support the concept that relief of pain with danazol is excellent and prolonged for many, but quite evanescent for women whose process seems to be only transiently affected by this form of therapy.

A dose study by Dmowski et al[98] is illuminating. Patients received danazol at 100, 200, 400 or 600mg daily for 6 months in a double-blind protocol. Laparoscopy before and after treatment, as well as a pelvic pain score was used to assess results. Improvement of pain scores, as well as the extent of amen-orrhea, were both related to the daily drug dose. At 100mg daily, pain scores had a 56% improvement, rising to 83% at the 600mg per day dose. But only half the patients became amenorrheic at the 600mg per day dose. These findings are in contradistinction to those reported by some other authors who claim that a daily dose of 400mg is sufficient. Generally speaking, patients with more advanced disease seem to require a full daily dose of 800mg for at least 6 months in order to achieve satisfactory control of their symptoms.

A similar study was done by Moore et al[99]. Minimal endometriosis responded to lower doses, but this was not true for the more advanced cases. Relief of pain, dysmenorrhea and dyspareunia occurred in 89%, but 51% had recurrence of symptoms within one year following completion of a 6 month course of therapy.

An excellent follow-up study was performed by Barbieri et al[100] who evaluated 100 patients over a mean of 49 months following treatment with 800 mg of danazol for varying durations, but with a mean of 17.3 weeks of therapy. In this older study, 57% had a laparotomy following pharmacologic therapy.

- Symtomatic improvement was reported by 89% (pre-surgery).
- 94% actually had reduced endometriotic involvement at the second look laparotomy or laparoscopy.
- But the overall recurrence rate was 33% during the follow-up interval.

Side effects included:

- Weight Gain
- Edema
- Decreased breast size
- Seborrhea and acne
- Hirsutism
- Voice deepening

As with many such studies, methodologic problems as well as patient compliance limit interpretation of the data. First, when comparing different reports, the mix of patients according to disease severity may be a problem. The disease process may have been existant for a longer period of time, and patients in one group may have had greater exposure to previous therapies. Patients who drop out of studies may do so for a variety of reasons with side-effects being one, but lack of therapeutic results another. Proper statistical methods must be employed to deal with this factor. Doses vary as with the studies reported herein, and treatment intervals are rarely uniform. Most studies with second look laparoscopy perform that procedure immediately following pharmacologic therapy in order to assess a drug effect, but the subsequent status of the patients often remains in doubt. In all fairness, patient compliance becomes a limiting bias later on; asymptomatic or pregnant patients may not cooperate in having a second look endoscopy, which leaves a group of symptomatic and infertile patients as the population generating the statistics of a second look procedure.

Puleo and Hammond[101] succeeded in evaluating a group of 39 women with a mean of 16.9 months of follow-up after completion of a 7.3 (mean) month course of danazol 800mg daily. Duration of treatment was proportional to the extent of the disease process seen at the initial laparoscopy.

- Relief of symptoms was noted by 97% (38/39) within 6 months of starting therapy.

- Advanced disease initially was associated with an increased chance of early exacerbation.

- Recurrent dysmenorrea was found in 38% (15/39) with ten having subsequent surgery (2 had hysterectomy and bilateral salpingo-oophrectomy).Symptoms recurred at a mean of 6.9 months, but were related to the initial staging.

An Italian study[102] compared the results of 600mg daily of danazol for endometriosis with

27mg daily of cyproterone acetate (CPA) a 17-OH progesterone derivative which has anti-gonadotropic, antiandrogenic and progestational activity. The CPA was given in conjunction with 0.035mg of ethinyl estradiol (EE) daily. 23 patients were randomly allocated to one or the other study group following laparoscopic verification and staging of endometriosis.

- After 6 months of treatment dysmenorrhea had disappeared in all.
- 6 months following completion of treatment, pain recurred in 66% of the CPA group and 58% of danazol patients. Comparable figures at one year were 89 % and 92%, respectively.
- Intermenstrual pelvic pain, initially dramatically improved in both groups, was found to be present in four patients in each group at 6 months and in all but one danazol subject after one year.
- Deep dyspareunia recurred by 6 months in all ten women with that complaint.
- As in other studies, except for an absent LH surge at mid-cycle, danazol patients had unchanged gonadotropins.
- CPA was more effective in lowering E2 levels, and all those patients became amenorrheic, but only 8/12 of the danazol patients achieved total amenorrhea.
- Menses resumed in 3-9 days after halting CPA versus 23-47 days following cessation of danazol.

- CPA was better tolerated than danazol.

- Acne and seborrhea actually improved on CPA, probably as a consequence of its antiandrogenic activity coupled with the accompanying EE.

This study suggests that CPA was as therapeutic for control of endometriosis associated pelvic pain as danazol. The drug, CPA, has been available in Europe for many years and has gained widespread acceptance as an antiandrogenic agent frequently used to control symptoms associated with polycystic ovarian syndrome. It has a good track record for safety and tolerance, and would appear to be efficacious for this indication as well.

MEGESTROL ACETATE

This agent known as Megace (Megestrol-acetate - Bristol Myers Squibb) is a progestin frequently used to treat carcinoma of the breast and/or endometrium. A study by Schlaff et al[103] examined the effect of 40mg daily in a group of 29 women having failed to improve after pre-vious therapies of various sorts for endometrio-sis. In general, pain relief by two months was excellent, but 10 of the 29 dropped out of therapy by four months because of lack of improvement or side effects of the usual progestational variety. This was a pilot study designed to establish an effective dose and to check tolerance. One might consider this approach in patients who refuse surgery and who have been unsuccessful with other pharmacological therapies. Megace has a good safety record with respect to serious side-effects.

GESTRINONE≠

Gestrinone is a synthetic trienic 19-nortestosterone steroid with antigonadotropic properties which binds to progesterone receptors. Moreover, the drug acts as an antiestrogen without actually binding to estrogen receptors. It has had clinical trials as an oral and intradermal contraceptive agent. Coutinho[104] treated a group of women with endometriosis and reported results in 20 who completed two years of follow-up after 6-8 months of therapy using 5mg orally taken twice weekly. More severe cases received the longer treatment protocol.

- Except for one patient with severe disease, all patients were free of dyspareunia by the second month and had no symptoms by three months.

- Acne, seborrhea, weight gain and hoarseness were the chief (androgenic) side-effects.

≠(Roussel-Uclaf, France)

Another gestrinone study was reported by Venturini et al[105]. This group used 2.5mg orally twice weekly in a small group of 11 patients with endometriosis. Mean endometriosis scores as assessed before and after therapy by laparoscopy were 17.2 and 9.1 after 6 months, respectively. Again, patients were essentially pain free by two months. But adverse lipid profile changes were encountered, probably as a consequence of its slightly androgenic action and the mechanism of displacing testosterone from its serum binding site. Gonadotropin and serum E_2 levels were unchanged from normal early follicular phase levels, but the antiestrogenic activity was thought to be the result of the drug's action to deplete the cytosol estrogen receptors and further to inhibit receptor recycling.

Given the androgenic side-effects, it seems unlikely that the French manufacturer of this drug will attempt to have it approved in North America since it has a clinical profile similar to that of danazol.

GONADOTROPIN RELEASING HORMONE AGONIST (GnRH-a)

(Also see discussion in Chapter 20)

The native GnRH is secreted in packets released at 90 minute or so intervals from the hypothalamus with a very short serum half life. When given exogenously as a continuous infusion, pituitary down-regulation or suppression occurs as documented brilliantly by the work of Schally's group and by the elegant monkey experiments by Knobil. Substitution at the six position of this decapeptide allows for protection from enzymatic degradation and substitution at the distal end of the molecule confers increased potency.

These agonists first stimulate, transiently, and then suppress pituitary release of FSH, and to a lesser degree LH, causing a clinical pseudomenopause. Pure antagonists were associated in clinical trials with unacceptably severe reaction to histamine release. Newer antagonists have been biodesigned to avoid this problem, but to date have a much shorter duration of pituitary suppression than the agonists which have been in actual clinical use. The agonists have opened up a number of exciting investigational avenues of pharmacologic treatment of various gynecologic conditions, including suppression of premature menarche, preoperative shrinkage of myoma uteri, the potential for long term therapy of both endometriosis and myoma, and pituitary control (suppression) during superovulation induction cycles, and palliation of premenstrual syndrome.

Leuprolide acetate (LA) was the first agonist approved in the United States for non-gynaecologic clinical use, with the indication being that of therapy for metastatic prostate carcinoma, i.e., to eliminate testicular production of testosterone. Nafarelin acetate (Synarel-Syntex) was the first GnRH-a approved for a gynaecologic indication, i.e., endometriosis, in the United States and Canada and remains, at the time of writing, the only agonist approved for this indication in Canada. Because of the European experience with various preparations of this sort, the North American gynaecologic community quickly adopted it for the indications mentioned above. The initial dose form was via a subcutaneous route for LA, and injections of 0.5mg were used once or twice daily to cause eventual pituitary suppression. A depot form followed, first with a 7.5mg monthly dose, and then with a 3.75mg monthly dose which has proven to be quite sufficient to cause profound pseudo-menopausal status in most, but not all, patients[3].

Nafarelin acetate is administered intranasally employing a metered nasal spray system at a dosage of 400-800 μg/day (each spray contains 200 μg nafarelin acetate).

Actually, that is one of the limiting features of therapy; namely, that estrogen levels are so low that vasomotor symptoms and the propensity for bone loss become clinical problems with prolonged use. Experimental programs of low dose estrogen replacement (give-back) and progestational supplementation seem to be able to solve these problems without blunting the therapeutic effect, provided that the proper agent and dose are chosen.

- Dysmenorrhea was milder ($p < 0.001$) at monthly visit 1-3 and on the final visit compared with placebo-treated patients.

- At the final visit dysmenorrhea was present in 7% versus the initial 96% of LA-treated patients and in 95% of the original 100% in the placebo group.

- Non-menstrual pain was present initially in all but two LA patients. This improved compared with the placebo group. Moreover, LA patients showed a cumulative improvement in reduction of pain with time.

- Dyspareunia was difficult to assess because of infrequent sexual activity in the study groups.

- Pelvic tenderness in general behaved similarly to that of pelvic pain. The latter, of course,is purely a patient subjective

TABLE 5
PELVIC PAIN SCORING SYSTEM.

Symptom	Grade	Description
Dysmenorrhea	Severe	In bed $\geq$ 1 d, incapacitation
	Moderate	In bed part of day, occasional loss of work
	Mild	Some loss of work efficiency
Dyspareunia	Severe	Avoids intercourse because of pain
	Moderate	Intercourse painful to the point of causing interdiction
	Mild	Tolerated discomfort
Pelvic Pain	Severe	Requiring strong analgesics. Persistent during cycle other than during menstruation
	Moderate	Noticeable discomfort for most of cycle
	Mild	Occassional pelvic discomfort
Pelvic tenderness	Severe	Unable to palpate because of tenderness
	Moderate	Extensive tenderness of palpation
	Mild	Minimal tenderness on palpation
Induration	Severe	Nodular adnexa and cul-de-sac, uterus frequently frozen
	Moderate	Thickened and indurated adnexa and cul-de-sac, restricted uterine mobility
	Mild	Uterus freely mobile, induration in the cul-de-sac

From Dlugi AM, Miller JD, Knittle J, Lupron Study Group: Lupron depot (leuprolide acetate for depot suspension) in the treatment of endometriosis : a randomized, placebo-controlled, double-blind study. Fertil Steril 54:419, 1990. Reprinted with permission of the publisher, The American Fertility Society.

TABLE 6
REDUCTION OF PAIN SCORES AFTER THERAPY FOR ENDOMETRIOSIS WITH DEPOT LUPRON.

	Lupron depot		Placebo		
Monthly visit	No.	Mean change	No.	Mean change	Between group
Dysmenorrhea					
1	28	-1.5	20	-0.3	$P < 0.001$
2	28	-2.4	20	-0.2	$P < 0.001$
3	28	-2.3	20	-0.3	$P < 0.001$
4	28	-2.4	6	-0.4	
5	28	-2.1	6	-0.5	
6	23	-2.0	1	-1.0	
Final	28	-2.2	21	-0.2	$P < 0.001$
Pelvic pain					
1	28	-0.5	20	-0.3	$P < 0.005$
2	28	-1.1	20	-0.3	$P < 0.005$
3	28	-1.2	20	-0.2	$P < 0.005$
4	28	-1.4	6	-1.1	
5	28	-1.7	6	-0.6	
6	23	-0.4	1	-1.0	
Final	28	-1.2	21	-0.3	$P = 0.001$
Dyspareunia					
1	14	-0.3	13	-0.2	
2	11	0	12	-0.2	
3	14	-0.2	13	0.1	
4	13	0	2	-0.6	
5	13	-0.1	2	-0.6	
6	12	-0.1	1	-1.0	
Final	17	-0.4	13	0.1	NS[a]
Pelvic tenderness					
1	26	-0.4	18	-0.1	NS
2	24	-0.7	18	-0.3	NS
3	27	-0.9	20	-0.3	$P = 0.005$
4	24	-1.0	6	-0.8	
5	26	-1.0	6	-0.6	
6	23	-1.6	1	-2.0	
Final	28	-1.0	21	-0.3	$P = 0.001$

[a] NS, not significant.

From Dlugi AM, Miller JD, Knittle J, Lupron Study Group: Lupron depot (leuprolide acetate for depot suspension) in the treatment of endometriosis : a randomized, placebo-controlled, double-blind study. Fertil Steril 54:419, 1990. Reprinted with permission of the publisher, The American Fertility Society.

analysis, while the former is an evaluation which is shared with the examiner.

- Pelvic induration scores had changes which were parallel to those of pelvic tenderness.

- Menses eventually were suppressed in all LA patients, but that effect was delayed in 10 of 27; 7 had one menses following the initial injection. Two patients appeared to escape from suppression after 60 days.

- Spotting during therapy was reported at least once by 17 of 27 LA patients (63%).

- Mean serum E_2 value for the LA group was < 30pg/ml (90pmol/l) but the two patients mentioned above had values in excess of 70 pg/ml (210 pmol/l).

- Dual photon absorptiometry in 15 LA patients showed a 3.6% decrease in spinal bone mineral density from baseline to the end of therapy at 6 months.

- Of interest was the finding of vasomotor episodes in 78% of the LA patients and in fully 29% of placebo patients. Flushes usually were rated as mild or moderate.

- Other adverse events in LA patients were headaches (34%), vaginitis, sweating, nausea, dizziness, and insomnia, all noted in 16% of the patients.

- A one year follow-up of 24 LA patents revealed 57% with recurrent dysmenorrhea at 6 months following completion of therapy. For patients starting with moderate to severe pelvic pain, 54% had returned to baseline pain levels by three months post-treatment.

- Fully 75% with dyspareunia had reduced discomfort at one year.

- Pelvic tenderness could not be elicited in 58% at one year who initially had that finding.

- Pelvic induration was not felt until the one year follow-up visit (none was noted at six months) and this was a finding in 33%.

- Six of eight with reduced bone density diagnosed by quantitative computer tomography at the end of therapy had normalized at one year. Loss was 11.8% of trabecular spinal bone diagnosed with this technique, compared with a loss of 2.2% for placebo patients.

- Slight elevations in LDL cholesterol were seen. The placebo group had a slight increase in prothrombin time, while the treated group had a slight decrease.

A large multicentric study was undertaken with the GnRH-a nafarelin (Synarel-Syntex) given as a twice daily nasal spray[107]. Two dose ranges were evaluated - a 400 ug and an 800 ug per day - and a double-blind protocol against 800 mg daily of danazol was used; i.e. patients had both spray and capsules, but only one was active. No surgical intervention was allowed at the time of the screening laparoscopy, since this would bias the results. The first report of this group dealt with 213 patients who completed 6 months of therapy including a second look laparoscopy.

Figure 15 shows the laparoscopic staging pre- and post-drug therapy for the three groups; no differences are noted in pre-treatment severity or in improvement following drug therapy.

Pain scores were tabulated according to dysmenorrhea, pain independent of menses, dyspareunia, and tenderness and induration during examination on a 0-3 scale, for a possible total of 15 points. Figure 16 details alterations in pain during 6 months of therapy according to initial AFS stage. Both agents demonstrated rapid and sustained pain relief in the majority of patients.

Table 6 shows the change in clinical symptoms in greater detail. Note that **worsening** during therapy was noted in all three groups in a small number of patients - 3 to 6% (the danazol excess is not of significant difference). The spectrum of change extended to apparent complete remission **soon after completion of therapy.**

Figure 17 shows the striking difference in effect of nafarelin versus danazol on lipro-proteins. Use of the nafarelin had no significant effect whereas danazol produced the expected androgenic adverse response of elevation of LDL and suppression of HDL levels.

Nafarelin patients sustained greater vasomotor symptoms and had more decrease in libido. This may be a net result of androgenic activity of danazol with displacement of serum testosterone from its binding site ameliorating somewhat vasomotor activity and offsetting the libido decrease apparently arising from reduction of estrogen levels. Edema and weight gain were greater, as expected, with use of danazol. Seborrhea and hirsutism, a priori, would have been expected to be higher with danazol based on prior experience, but this was not observed.

Very similar results were attained by Rolland and van der Heijden[108] in 194 patients in a 13 center European study utilizing nafarelin 400 ug/day versus danazol 400mg daily.

Leuprolide acetate as a 3.75mg IM depot form (Lupron, depot; TAP/Abbott) was given in a randomized double-blind placebo protocol in 52 patients with endometriosis over a 20 week interval.[106] If no relief was noted by 12 weeks, the code could be broken, and placebo patients could then be switched to active drug, but these patients were not included in this particular report. Second look laparoscopy and/or pelvic pain scoring system (Table 5) were used to assess results.

Table 6 shows the results of that study in which the numbers signify a reduction of pain scores.

SUMMARY

Medical therapy for endometriosis-associated pain using GnRH-a is approved for 6

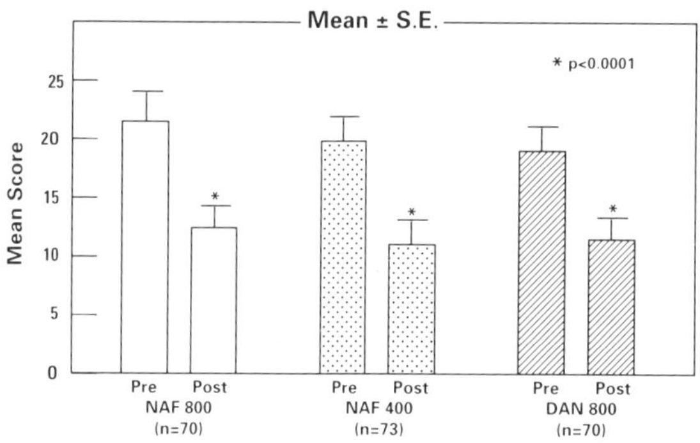

Fig. 15 From Henzl MR, Corson SL, Moghissi K et al: Administration of nasal nafarelin as compared with oral danazol for endometriosis. N Eng J Med 318:485, 1988. Reproduced with permission of the publisher.

months of use. Danazol is limited to a 9 month course by most. Metabolically, danazol produces an adverse lipid profile, and may also have negative effects on hepatic enzymatic studies; the GnRH-a are associated with reduction of bone mineral content of approximately 1% per month of use. Judicious use of history and physical examination allows the physician to choose the medication best suited to the individual patient, with special consideration given to family cardiovascular history, patient lipid profile, and skeletal type. Bone demineralization seems to be promptly reversible in most patients, and theoretically, supplementation with low-dose estrogen and/or progestin may allow for stabilization of bone without reduction of therapeutic effect. Two recent studies address this issue[109,110]. The study by

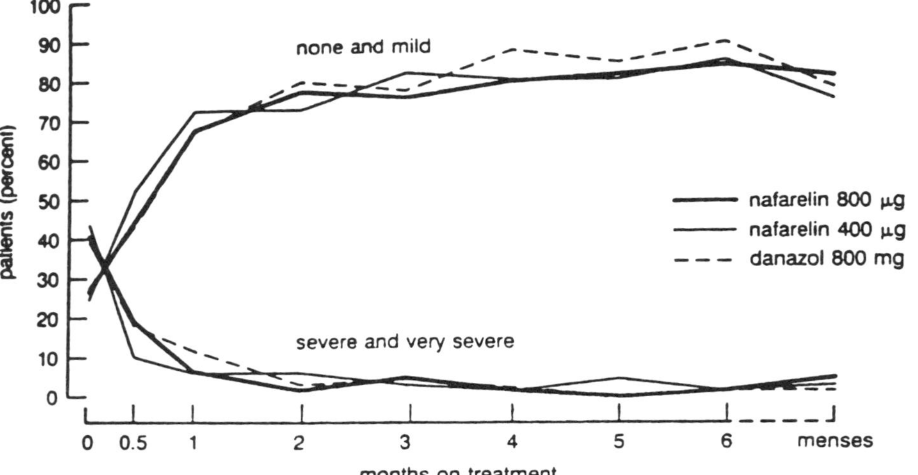

Fig. 16 Relief of symptoms in patients taking nafarelin or danazol for endometriosis. Note rapidity and maintenance of improvement. From Henzl MR, Corson SL, Moghissi K et al: Administration of nasal nafarelin as compared with oral danazol for endometriosis. N Eng J Med 318:485, 1988. Reproduced with permission of the publisher.

Surrey et al[110], in particular, showed that addition of norethindrone to GnRH-a therapy for endometriosis had no effect on estrogen levels, pain relief, or indices of bone metabolism. Another method of dealing with iatrogenic production of osteoporosis is to combine analog therapy with two weeks of disphosphonate administration given at 15 week intervals with the benefit accruing primarily from osteoclastic inhibition. In reviewing the literature on medical therapy of endometriosis-associated pain reasonable conclusions are:

- The vast majority of patients have significant reduction of pain within two months, although onset is slower with MPA and symptoms initially worsen when oral contraceptives are used.

NAFARELIN FOR ENDOMETRIOSIS

HIGH AND LOW DENSITY LIPOPROTEINS

Mean of Percent Changes from Baseline at End of 6-Months Treatment

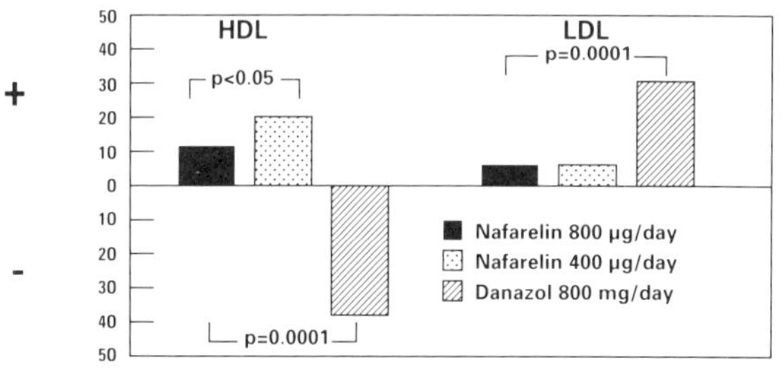

Fig. 17 From Henzl MR, Corson SL, Moghissi K et al: Administration of nasal nafarelin as compared with oral danazol for endometriosis. N Eng J Med 318:485, 1988. Reproduced with permission of the publisher.

TABLE 4

CHANGES IN SEVERITY: RELIEF OF CLINICAL SYMPTOMS OF ENDOMETRIOSIS

Treatment	No. of patients	Complete relief		Partial relief		No change		Worsened	
		No.	%	No.	%	No.	%	No.	%
Study I									
NAF800	70	38	54	27	39	3	4	2	3
NAF400	73	34	47	33	45	2	3	4	5
DAN800	70	34	49	29	41	3	4	4	6

NAF800, Nafarelin, 800 µg/day (400 µgtwice a day); *NAF400*, nafarelin, 400 µG/day (200 µg twice a day); *DAN800*, danazol, 800 mg/day (400 mg twice a day); *DAN600*, danazol, 600 mg/day (200 mg three times a day).

From Henzl MR, Kwei L[267]

- With all forms of treatment some patients will not experience improvement. This may be a function of implants failing to respond because of loss or alteration of enzyme systems or inadequate levels of drug delivery to the lesions.

- By one year following completion of therapy about half of the patients who had a good response will relapse to a level sufficient to affect their sense of well being. Whether this is because of exacerbation of preexisting, inadequately-treated lesions or development of new implants is conjectural, but probably represents both. Other patients have prolonged remission. Therapy is on a trial or emperic basis, since no markers for success have been identified as a pretherapeutic test.

- Annoying side effects may be seen with all therapeutic choices. Most are not acutely of great importance, except the hepatic enzymatic changes seen with danazol. None of the therapies has been associated, for instance, with an increase in embolic phenomenon, even with the high dose contraceptive agents. Nevertheless the long-term sequelae of repeated therapies causing changes in lipoprotein profiles and bone demineralization must be investigated.

#14 SURGICAL TREATMENT OF ENDOMETRIOSIS-ASSOCIATED PAIN

Presacral neurectomy (PSN)

Relief of pain centers about removal or ablation of endometriotic implants. Beyond that, pelvic pain can be managed with a number of surgical approaches to interruption of afferent sensory nerve pathways.

Pain which is central rather than lateral tends to be conveyed by afferent fibers entering the spinal cord at levels from L-1 to T-10. These fibers which service the uterus and proximal fallopian tube, eventually form the superior hypogastric plexus, known as the presacral nerve. In most cases this is a loose bundle of two or three partially fused trunks of nerve fibers rather than a single definable structure. The plexus lies retroperitoneally, centrally located around the mid-line at the level of L4-L5 just above the middle sacral artery and vein which rest on the vertebral periosteum. Fibers pass downward via the inferior hypogastric plexus to enter the uterosacral ligaments and over the rectal ampulla to Frankenhäuser's plexus. Retroperitoneal structures in the vicinity of the presacral nerve which must be identified during surgery include the aorta and iliac arteries, the vena cava and its tributaries, the right ureter (always) and often the left, and the inferior mesenteric blood vessels.

Details of surgical technique can be found in appropriate surgical texts. In brief, the posterior peritoneum is opened and the nervous tissue is dissected free of the areolar tissue and swept medially from both sides as the ureter is retracted laterally. The colon needs to be retracted laterally in order to gain exposure. The nerve bundle is then tied off in two locations and cut between the ligature. The operation was popularized in America after a positive review by Black[111] who reported on 9,937 cases in the world's literature in which relief from dysmenorrhea was in the 70%-80% range. An excellent discussion appears in an article by Malinak[112] in which he emphasizes the ability of the procedure to offer relief from deep dyspareunia, dysmenorrhea and sacral backache. Presecaral neurectomy is rarely performed in the absence of other endometriosis-related procedures.

PSN has had an uneven geographic distribution, being more popular in certain areas in the Southwest than others. For instance, Polan and DeCherney[113] reported on only 20 patients over a 7 year interval in New Haven, of whom only 8 had endometriosis. Relief was documented at 2.3 years following surgery with 75% still pain-free. A control group having pelvic surgery for pain but without PSN had a 25% continued relief from pain at 3.5 years following surgery. As with other studies, there was no correlation between pain relief and subsequent fertility when presacral neurectomy was performed. Previously, Garcia and David[114] reported relief of dyspareunia in 74% and elimination of dysmenorrhea in 97% following PSN.

Lee et al[115] studied results of PSN with and without accompanying resection of the uterosacral ligaments; no difference in pain relief was noted. Followup in 45 patients over 31 months was achieved. Dysmenorrhea was relieved in 73% and dyspareunia improved in 77%, 19 were pain free, but five had no change. Forty-five initially improved, and eight (18%) subsequently developed lateral pelvic pain which necessitated further surgery in four. This pain recurred at 19 months on average, and was usually associated with involvement of the ovaries by endometriosis. One patient sustained major blood loss during PSN secondary to laceration of a middle sacral blood vessel. Another had permanent mild impairment of urinary function post-operatively, but this has been a rare complication in the literature.

Beginning in the decade of 1970 operative laparoscopy, first with electrosurgery, and then with lasers, became a popular alternative to laparotomy for surgical intervention in endometriosis, and PSN became rarely performed. Perez[116], however, has described a laparoscopic approach to PSN. Preliminary results were good. As with other studies, subsequent development of lateral pelvic pain heralded development of adnexal endometriosis.

Laparoscopic Uterine Nerve Ablation (LUNA)

Doyle in 1955[117] found that 70% of patients having interruption of the uterosacral ligaments (performed vaginally) reported pain relief. Lichten and Bombard [118] studied a group of 21 patients not achieving pain relief with a combination of non-steroidal anti-inflammatory drugs (NSAIDs) and oral contraceptive agents. In a small but well-controlled study, benefit of the LUNA procedure was documented, but also a decreased efficacy over time was noted. Our own experience is that with endometriosis, the LUNA procedure gives good results when lesions are present in the posterior pelvic compartment and especially when the uterosacral ligaments are involved. As with PSN, results are poor when pain has a lateral distribution. In our own series of 242 patients with endometriosis who complained of pain, use of the YAG laser with a sapphire probe laparoscopically for ablation of lesions and LUNA for posterior pelvic disease has brought about complete relief of pain in 72% at one year, and satisfactory response to NSAIDs in another 16% at one year. By 17 months, these results were reduced to 57% and 11%, respectively.

Principles of Conservative Endometriosis Surgery

Now that enthusiasm for laparoscopic techniques has become widespread, instrumentation has improved, and the net result is that the tenants for conservative endometriosis surgery do not differ between laparotomy and laparoscopy.

- All visible disease should be erradicated by removal, vaporization, or in situ destruction.

- Biopsy, particularly of ovarian cystic lesions

and of any suspicious area should be performed prior to application of energy.

- Preoperative CA 125 levels and ultrasonic assessment of adnexal masses are helpful.

- Septation, irregular contour, apparent papillation, and/or solid components seen ultrasonographically within an ovarian cyst should be considered as indicative of ovarian pathology other than endometriosis.

- At the time of surgery, a thorough examination of the peritoneal cavity and close inspection of the ovarian lesion should be performed prior to entry into the cyst. Excresences denote neoplastic disease. These may sometimes be safely biopsied on the surface of the lesion without entry.

- Adhesions are frequently present prior to surgery because of a brisk inflammatory response. Preoperative use of medical therapy (to be discussed later) may be helpful. If such a great inflammatory response is unexpectedly encountered, one may wish to employ a course of medical therapy prior to definitive surgery.

- Adhesions are best cut at both ends and removed.

- "Meticulous" reperitonealization favored as a microsurgical technique may be counte-rproductive in that ischemia caused by placing tissue on stretch plus the effect of suture may cause more, rather than fewer adhesions to form.

- The role of adjuvants to prevent adhesion formation is not yet clear.

- There is no consensus that laser surgery, per se, is any better than skillfully employed mechanical or electrosurgical techniques. Lasers, however, do permit destruction of lesions juxtaposed to sensitive structures such as bowel, bladder and ureter.

Nezhat et al[119] compared CO_2, Argon and KTP/532 lasers, and concluded that the CO_2 laser was slightly superior for both pain relief and restoration of fertility in endometriosis. Keye et al[120] reported 92% of 50 women had reduction of pain after argon laser surgery.

- I personally view six hour, or longer, laparoscopic procedures to excise the posterior cul-de-sac, peritoneum, and most of the recto-vaginal septum free of **visible** implants as folly. These patients obviously have a systemic rather than a localized process, which requires pharmacologic therapy. Debulking procedures, as with oncologic disease, must be guided by sound surgical judgment.

- **A warmed** irrigant used in generous quantities is central to good technique. My own preference is lactated Ringers with 5000U of heparin and 1:600,000 dilution of epinephrine per liter. High pressure irrigators

(Corson Aspirator/Irrigator-Cabot Medical) can facilitate development of tissue cleavage planes.

- Adhesions to ovaries cause pain often greater than that encountered with endometriosis alone. Reformation is always a problem especially on the left from the mesocolon. Light electrodessication or laser treatment of surface endometriosis and adhesions is useful. **Perhaps** the newer barrier agents may help.

- Appendectomy should be performed if the appendix is involved, and is advocated by some as a routine prophylactic measure.

- Drainage of ovarian endometriomas alone seems to be insufficient to prevent reformation, although some dissent.[121] Ovarian endometriomas can be treated by stripping the cyst wall, vaporization or coagulation dependent on the anatomy and one's surgical preference.

- We do not believe in application of suture to the ovary. Hemostasis can be achieved with the YAG laser or by electrosurgical means. Regardless of suture type, the best suture in the ovary is none at all. The edges collapse on themselves after the endometrioma has been drained, and second-look laparoscopy has demonstrated excellent healing with no or minimal adhesion formation.

- An ovary which apears to be hopelessly damaged reproductively often has compressed normal stroma between the cyst wall and the ovarian tunic. When oophorectomy is necessary, the newer laparoscopic instruments such as the Multifire Endo GIA 30- Stapler (Autosuture-United States Surgical Corp.) make the procedure quite easy.

A number of authors have published on laparoscopic oophorectomy [122-125] using a variety of techniques. Maiman et al[126] discussed the issue of malignant neoplasms thought to be benign treated laparoscopically. In our own experience, frozen section diagnosis has been very helpful.

- Uterine suspension should be employed judiciously, and then only when extreme retroversion is found in conjunction with posterior disease. We favor a temporary suspension since use of permanent suture can lead to kinking of the proximal tube and (rarely) to internal herniation of the bowel through a small median aperture between the suspended round ligament and the anterior abdominal wall.

- Uterosacral plication can form a shelf on which ovaries can rest, separated from raw posterior cul-de-sac tissue. This is often helpful, but over zealous advancement of the ligaments towards the midline can cause ureteral compromise by kinking or actual suture placement.

- Uterosacral interruption should be performed medially as to safeguard the ureter, and a depth of 3-5mm is sufficient. The YAG laser's hemostatic properties are helpful since arterial bleeding from a deep vessel may be encountered. The results are the same regardless of whether a laser, electrosurgical, or mechanical means are employed.

- Actual endometriosis within the uterosacral ligament may be deeper than 4mm, but can be destroyed with laser or electrosurgical techniques. Bipolar coagulation may be insufficient.

- Deep involvement of the colon may necessitate resection and anastomosis, preceded by colonoscopy, barium enema and a bowel preparation. Laparoscopic techniques for bowel resection are still experimental.

- Efficacy of second-look procedures, primarily for control of adhesions is still not clear.

The Final Solution

Unfortunately, in spite of sensible programs of management and well-performed surgery, some patients will have a progressive course leading to incapacitation with daily pain. When hysterectomy is performed, remember that it is estrogen which seems to be most important in fueling the activity of the implants. Surgically, I believe that it is incongruous to leave ovarian tissue when hysterectomy is performed for pain associated with endometriosis. Moreover, it makes little or no sense to institute full estrogen replacement in the immediate post-operative interval. Instead, our practice is to give MPA as a 200mg injection at three month intervals for 12-18 months to treat residual implants along the vaginal cuff and elsewhere in the pelvis. This also controls vasomotor symptoms. Then estrogen therapy is cautiously initiated with pelvic examination at regular intervals over the next year to rule out stimulation of any residual endometriosis.

Too often I have seen patients referred for post hysterectomy pain who received immediate estrogen replacement, or who had not had total ovarian extirpation. These patients have been found to have active endometriosis in the bowel, bladder, and along the vaginal cuff. Surgery and/or prolonged pharmacologic therapy has been necessary to control symptoms.

ENDOMETRIOSIS

1.	Definition	Presentation Classification and Diagnosis
2.	Morphology	
3.	Etiologies	
4.	Prevalence & Heredity	
5.	Clinical Presentation and Symptoms	
6.	Clinical Signs	
7.	Diagnostic Studies	
8.	Differential Diagnosis	
9.	Malignant Transformation	
10.	Classification	
11.	Peritoneal	Anatomic Distribution
12.	Extra Abdominal Extra Pelvic	
13.	Medications	Pain and its Therapy
14.	Surgery	

ENDOMETRIOSIS

#15 INFERTILITY HORMONAL CHANGES

Figure 18 illustrates some of the mechanisms by which endometriosis may exert an adverse effect on fertility. It should not be surprising that if diagnosis is often difficult, choice of therapy is even more confusing with the spectrum running from no active treatment for minimal disease, through medication and conservative surgery, to hysterectomy with castration for advanced cases. Combinations of medical and surgical approaches are often employed in either order.

Most intriguing is the issue of why some women with seemingly minimal endometriosis have persistent infertility. Is this merely a coincidence? If cause and effect, then what are the mechanisms involved? Can some simple serum marker be identified as prognostic for future fertility? What do the seemingly minor changes noted in some hormonal studies and in peritoneal fluid content mean? Are these changes like a pack of dominoes; is there a fixed order to the cascade as with the clotting factors?

In this section some of the alterations of normal homeostasis found in patients with endometriosis will be discussed. Well-designed and properly performed studies not infrequently have given divergent data. There are no hormonal changes specifically associated with endometriosis, and alterations noted may be chance occurrences rather than related findings.

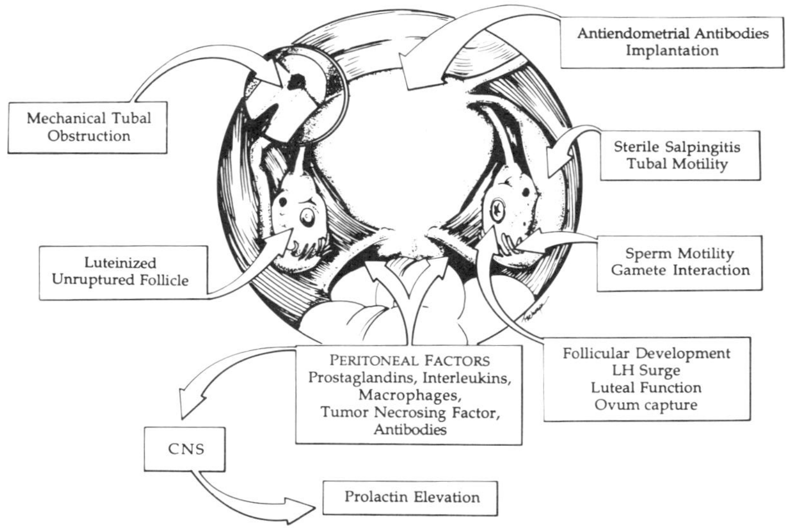

Antiendometrial Antibodies
Implantation

Mechanical Tubal
Obstruction

Sterile Salpingitis
Tubal Motility

Luteinized
Unruptured Follicle

Sperm Motility
Gamete Interaction

PERITONEAL FACTORS
Prostaglandins, Interleukins,
Macrophages,
Tumor Necrosing Factor,
Antibodies

Follicular Development
LH Surge
Luteal Function
Ovum capture

CNS

Prolactin Elevation

Fig. 18. Mechanisms of Infertility Associated with Endometriosis

Prolactin Effect

Muse et al[127] described elevated prolactin (PRL) concentrations in serum in infertile women with endometriosis versus fertile controls (infertile women without endometriosis would have been a good choice as a third group). The mean values, however, were not statistically different. But with thyroid releasing hormone (TRH) stimulation, augmented values of PRL were almost twice those of the controls, and were increased proportionately to the stage of the disease. Haney et al[128] measured peritoneal PRL since PRL is known to be produced by luteal phase endometrium. No difference was found compared with fertile controls and women infertile with tubal or adhesive disease. But the weight of other studies [129-131] would indicate that patients with endometriosis do not have disordered PRL metabolism, and patients with both pathologic entities have coincident problems.

Periovulatory and Luteal Phase Dysfunction

The delicate sequence of events occurring just before physical ovulation sets the stage for luteal phase function. The rate of rise of E_2 may be just as important as the peak levels obtained. The temporal relationship between serum E_2, P and LH levels are like shadows on a wall, reflecting the tremendous rapid metabolic changes within the maturing follicle and pituitary release of LH. Any subtle disturbance might lead to a disordered ovulatory-luteal state. Cheeseman et al[132] found two distinct midcycle peaks of LH, two or three days apart, in endometriosis patients as measured in daily early morning urine. Estriol-16-glucuronide secretion was delayed, and pregnanediol-3-glucuronide concentrations did not rise until the second peak. This functional shortening of luteal phase hormonal secretion may have been a consequence of a breakdown of normal hormonal feedback mechanisms. In a later work [133] this group postulated a delay in P secretion although midluteal levels were no different from controls. But other workers have concluded that these findings are no more common in endometriosis patients than in other infertile populations especially those with unexplained infertility or mild ovulatory defects.[134] The more recent studies, moreover, have had the advantage of serial ultrasonic study of follicular growth and apparent subsequent rupture. Acosta et al[51] found that 27% of 103 infertile endometriosis patients were anovulatory.

Soules et al [136] noted anovulation in 17% of 350 women with endometriosis. Dmowski et al[137] found that 24% of 1941 infertile women having laparoscopy had endometriosis, and that 10% were anovulatory. When ovulatory induction alone was given as the initial therapy (no endometriotic specific therapy), the pregnancy rate was 50%. Badawy et al[138] found that 5% of 103 laparoscopically proven cases of endometriosis who were infertile also had anovulation. Another 22% had oligoovulation or luteal phase dysfunction. Therefore, endometriosis, per se, especially when mild, does not seem to predispose to gross ovulatory defects more frequently than what is expected in the general infertile population.

Ronnberg et al[139] described reduced LH receptors in ovarian follicles and in corpora lutea in endometriosis patients during the follicular phase and in luteal phase studies. This finding might explain both disordered ovulation and subsequent luteal phase dysfunction. While ultrasonic studies usually are employed to investigate the luteinized unruptured follicle (LUF) syndrome, Doody et al[140] used this modality to demonstrate abnormal follicular growth in endometriosis patients with the abnormality uncorrected by administration of clomiphene citrate. Using hormonal analyses, ultrasound and laparoscopy, Tummon et al[141] concluded that subtle ovulatory defects in the temporal relationship between E_2 and LH were no different in endometriosis patients than other infertile women with unexplained infertility.

Two animal model studies are of interest. The first was conducted by Kaplan et al[142] in which ovarian endometriosis was induced in rabbits. Ovulation was observed in stimulated cycles, and the number of ovulation points was adversely affected by the extent of ovarian adhesions present. These results are of interest, and may relate to severe endometriosis but do not seem to explain infertility seen with mild disease.

The other study was that of Schenken et al[143] who found that impaired fertility in monkeys with induced endometriosis was accounted for by failure of follicular rupture (LUF) in moderate cases and pelvic adhesions in more severe disease.

Luteal phase defects (LPD) may be diagnosed by progesterone determinations, but endometrial biopsy remains the gold standard. The sole prospective study examining the effect of endometriosis on LPD was reported by Pittaway et al[144] in 68 patients with and 75 patients without endometriosis. LPD was found in 9% and 5%, respectively, (no statistical difference).

Luteinized Unruptured Follicle (LUF) Syndrome

Probably no topic has caused more controversy in luteal phase evaluation than this one, and especially as related to endometriosis. Dhont et al[145], among others, has shown clearly that serum hormonal assays are not diagnostic, and that either laparoscopic "evidence" of a stigma, or lack thereof, is flimsy at best. Peritoneal fluid hormonal assays are helpful because of the high steroidal content of follicular fluid that can be collected from the cul-de-sac shortly after actual ovulation. Endometrial biopsy, however, is not helpful in diagnosis of this entity. Serial ultrasonic examinations have emerged as the gold standard here. Diagnosis is usually made by continuing follicular size increase after the LH surge, with continued failure to show collapse and the appearance of internal echoes consistent with formation of a corpus luteum. Even so, I remember patients in our own practice who conceived during the cycle in which this diagnosis was made ultrasonographically. Studies in women over multiple cycles suggest that few patients experience LUF for more than an occasional episode.

In a selected group of 33 patents with unexplained infertility, in which LUF figured to be relatively common, Daly et al[146] found a prevalence of 9% by ultrasonography, and only 6% had similar findings in the subsequent cycle.

Neither the Dhont study nor that reported by Koninckx et al[147] found a difference in prevalence of LUF between infertile patients with and without endometriosis using assay of peritoneal fluid obtained laparoscopically.

But different results were reported by Liukkonen et al[148] using ultrasound (US) and laparoscopy/laparotomy for diagnosis. A much higher prevalence was found, and results were similar to those reported by Brosens et al[149] who found ovulatory stigmata in only 21% of endometriosis patients versus 94% of controls laparoscoped at a similar point in the cycle. Brosens also found a shortened interval from LH peak to menses and a delayed P rise in endometriosis patients. Donnez et al[150] correlated laparoscopic findings with peritoneal fluid studies, and found that when a stigma was not seen, P was < 30 ng/mL in 94% of cases versus a low P in 12% of fertile controls.

The picture here remains cloudy at best. We would like to believe that endometriosis with its accompanying PG abnormalities could induce an ovulatory defect and subsequent luteal phase disorder as a result of a pertubation if not a frank disruption of a delicate sequential hormonal process. But proof currently is circumstantial, at best.

#16 PERITONEAL FLUID STUDIES

The literature on peritoneal fluid (PF) and prostaglandin (PG) content vis a vis endometriosis is a confusing one, chiefly for two reasons.

- First, fluid volume and concentrations of the constituents of PF are dependent on stage of the menstrual cycle in which measurement is performed, and many studies have not controlled for this.

- Second, many different prostanoids may be measured; some are stable for only a matter of minutes, and values are greatly affected by contamination with blood.

Peritoneal Fluid Cell Content

Normally, PF contains leukocytes in concentrations of 0.5 to 2.0 x 10^6/mL of which 85% are macrophages[151]. These cells have origin in bone marrow, circulate as monocytes, and then migrate from the vascular compartment to various body cavities where they function primarily as phagocytes when activated. Haney et al[152] found that concentrations of macrophages were similar between controls and patients with endometriosis, but because of increased PF volume, total counts were higher for the latter group. Halme et al[153-154] studied patients with mild endometriosis and concluded:

- Much of the local effect of macrophage activity was a consequence of substances released by these cells.

- Staining for histochemical evidence of macrophage activity such as with acid phosphatase, showed 46% activation for endometriotic patients versus 15% activation for macrophages in controls.

- Actual macrophage concentration was unchanged.

- No difference in PG levels in PF were found versus fertile controls.

Badawy et al[155] conducted a similar study and concluded:

- PF content of acid phosphatase was higher for patients with endometriosis versus controls.

- Endometrial cell count was higher in PF for patients with endometriosis than controls.

- PGF_2 , PGE_2, and Complement C_{3c} and C_4 were increased in patients.

- Total macrophage count was higher for patients versus controls, but proportion of morphologically activated cells was the same allowing for cycle timing of PF collection.

In a later publication, Halme et al [156] examined the relationship between endometriosis and peritoneal macrophages on a cause and effect basis. Zeller et al[157] used chemiluminescence to document macrophage activity in PF of women with endometriosis.

A most interesting study was performed by Schenken and Asch[158] who created endometriosis in rabbits.

- Impaired fertility versus controls was demonstrated with ovulation failure a separate cause from adhesion formation.
- PF concentrations of PGF were increased.

Prostaglandin Studies

Moon et al[159] documented the presence of PGF in human endometriosis implants. Drake et al[160] measured stable metabolites of Thromboxane A_2 (TxA_2) and prostacyclin, finding that there was an increase over controls. They theorized that these mediators of smooth muscle contraction might cause infertility by altered tubal function, but cycle timing was not controlled. Drake's group[161] previously had suggested an increased PF value in endometriosis, but this study also was not cycle controlled. Figure 19 demonstrates common pathways of PG metabolism.

Badawy et al[162] could not demonstrate cycle dependent PF concentrations of PG's, nor were there differences between patients with unexplained infertility and those with endometriosis.

Dawood et al[163] laparoscopically examined patients with chronic pelvic pain, chronic pelvic inflammatory disease, endometriosis and normal controls. PF studies with cycle timing being

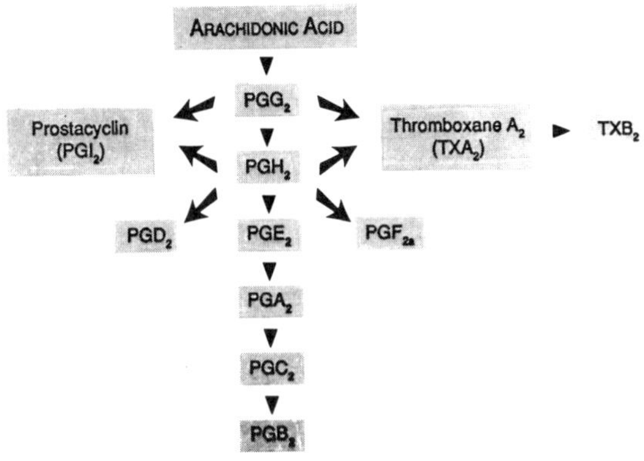

Fig. 19. Outline of common pathways of prostaglandin metabolism.

noted showed no difference for PG E_2, $PGF_{2\alpha}$ or Thromboxane B_2 (TxB_2). But 6-ketoprostaglandin F_1 (6-KF) was elevated in patients with endometriosis by concentration but was not statistically greater by total amount. PF volumes were similar in all groups. As an indicator of prostacyclin levels, the 6-KF metabolite might suggest tubal hypotonia but the data did not support that conclusion as an actuality.

Schenken et al[143] continued their animal studies, but used monkeys to demonstrate that induced endometriosis could cause infertility not only by formation of pelvic adhesions, but by production of luteal phase defect and because of unruptured luteinized follicles as well. Moderate and severe cases were associated with increased PF levels of PG $F_{2\alpha}$ with no change in PG E_2 noted.

Other PF constituents have been investigated. Eisermann et al[164] found an increase in tumor necrosis factor (TNF) in the PF of women with pelvic inflammatory disease and with moderate or severe endometriosis. Women who were nulligravid or nulliparous had higher values than those with two or more pregnancies-deliveries. TNF is secreted by activated macrophages and is cytotoxic to susceptible cells. This is another observation in the cascade of endometriosis-induced events. The actual sequence and cause and effect relationships are still to be elucidated.

Hill et al[165] used monoclonal antibodies rather than histologic morphology to identify cell types in PF. Women with **early** stages of endometriosis had the most significant elevations of total leukocytes, macrophages, helper T lymphocytes and natural killer cells. These findings support an active immunologic process which will be discussed separately.

About the time when controversy over PF volume in endometriosis seem to be at an ebb, Syrop and Halme[166] reported that PF volume showed an inverse relationship to occurrence of pregnancy in endometriosis patients who were followed for two years after laparoscopy. Mean fluid volume was 16.2 ml $\pm$1.1 SEM.

In general, PF volume increases through the proliferative phase, peaking at early secretory phase with a late luteal decline.[167-168] Rock was involved in two well designed studies of PF and endometriosis[169-170]. The first study was performed between cycle days 8-12. Laparoscopically obtained PF was measured and analyzed for PG metabolites. No PG elevation was noted compared with normals, and no relationship was found between the stage of endometriosis and any of the four prostanoids measured. No increase of PF volume could be shown for endometriotic patients. Later work from the same department[170] investigated women who had laparoscopy between cycle days 13-18. The results were as before in that no differences in volume or PG content compared with controls was found.

De Leon et al[171] found increases in PF volume, E_2, P and epidermal growth factor during the secretory phase versus the proliferative phase in all patients with no difference between normal controls and those with endometriosis. But while no change in PG's was found according to cycle timing, endometriotic patients had higher PG content primarily in the secretory phase. Kauma et al[172] documented that fibronectin, a growth factor for fibroblasts, was elaborated by activated macrophages within the peritoneal cavity, with approximately a threefold increase in production, but with a 30% lower concentration in peritoneal fluid, indicating a rapid metabolism. Thus, the activation of macrophages could be translated into elaboration of a marker for the inflammatory process. With respect to the cause and effect relationship, this could simply be a mechanism to help wall off an inflammatory process.

Joshi et al[173] described a unique protein present only in PF during the secretory phase in women with endometriosis but its importance beyond that of serving as a marker is yet unknown.

Given the presence of activated macrophages and PG's and PF, what are the ramifications for sperm interaction? In a landmark paper Muscato et al[174] demonstrated that peritoneal macrophages phagocytized sperm in vitro, and that cells from women with endometriosis showed a greater action (84%) against normal sperm than cells obtained from controls (43%). Chacho et al[175] extended the studies made on PF. No changes in prostanoids were found, but PF value, macrophage content and activation were all increased in patients with endometriosis. When sperm were exposed to incubated fluid containing macrophages, a decrease in hamster egg penetration assay scores were noted.

A good clinical study was done by Stone and Himsl[176] who inseminated patients just prior (2-4 hours) to laparoscopy and then collected cul-de-sac fluid. No difference in motile sperm numbers could be found according to presence or absence of mild endometriosis. Burke[177], however, reported reduced sperm velocity ***in vitro*** when PF in patients with endometriosis was added to the medium. Sueldo et al[178] reported that PF in general reduced fertilization of murine oocytes in vitro when added to the medium, but the effect was enhanced when PF from endometriosis patients was tested. Moreover, the factor was both filterable and heat labile. Conversely, Leach et al [179] using a computerized semen analysis system, found PF in patients with endometriosis had no effect on sperm velocity with up to 6 hours of incubation.

Steinleitner et al[180] investigated possible embryo toxic effects of PF in hamsters. PF from endometriotic patients, injected intra-peritoneally, caused a decreased in oocyte recovery and embryo development. The substance proved to be heat labile. Similarly, Prough et al[181] found that a heat labile substance in PF from endometriosis patients, obtained during follicular phase laparoscopy, did not promote growth of the two-cell mouse embryo system.

Sueldo et al[182] later evaluated human recombinant interleukin-1 (IL-1), an immuno-

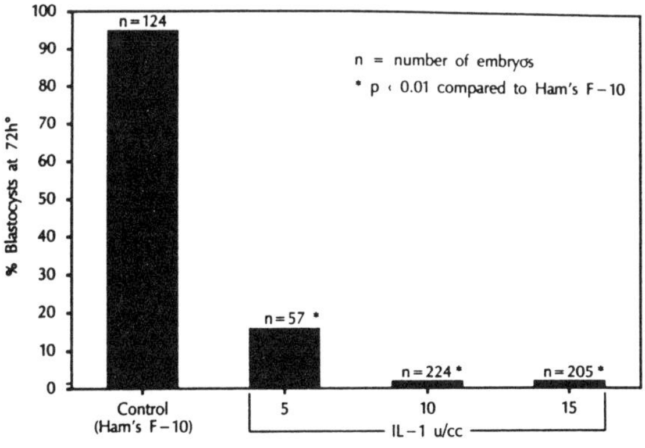

Fig. 20. Inhibition of blastocyst formation in the mouse embryo by interleuken-1.
From Sueldo CE, Kelly E, Montoro L, Subia E, Baccaro M, Swanson JA, Steinleitner A, Lambert H: Effect of Interleukin-1 on Gamete Interaction and Mouse Embryo Development, J Reprod Med 35:868, 1990. Reproduced with permission from the Journal of Reproductive Medicine.

TABLE 7
EFFECT OF HETEROLOGOUS MACROPHAGE TRANSFER ON EARLY REPRODUCTIVE EVENTS

	Unfertilized oocytes	4 - Cell embryos	Fertilization
Control (no macrophages transferred)	0	24.1 ± 3.4	100
Unstimulated macrophages	0.6 ± 0.3	23.9 ± 1.1	97.6 ± 1.0
Hyperactivated macrophages	19.8 ± 1.6	0.2 ± 0.3	0.9 ± 0.6
Ex vivo deactivated macrophages	2.4 ± 1.0	18.3 ± 1.6	93.8 ± 2.9
Erythrocytes	2.7 ± 1.5	17.7 ± 1.7	86.8 ± 7.3

From Steinleitner A, Lambert H, Lauredo I: Heterologous transplantation of activated murine peritoneal macrophages inhibits gamete interaction in vivo: a paradigm for endometriosis-associated subfertility. Fertil Steril 54:725, 1990.

active macrophage product, in the mouse embryo system. No change in sperm velocity was noted, but human sperm penetration in the hamster system was reduced by addition of IL-1 as was the zona pellucida assay. IL-1 significantly inhibited the development of the mouse embryos (Figure 20).

Steinleitner et al[183] in an elegant study, activated mice macrophages with thioglycolate and injected (IP) these cells as well as deactivated (with a protein synthesis inhibitor, emetine) cells and non-activated macrophages into ovarian stimulated mice about to be mated. Oocyte recovery and embryo recovery were both depressed by activated macrophages, but this effect was reversed by emetene, and was not seen with macrophages in the basal state. Table 7 demonstrates the dramatic effect. Embryo toxicity was also demonstrated in a study by Marcos et al[184].

Damewood et al[185] used a two-cell mouse embryo system to evaluate the effect of serum from patients with mild to moderate endometriosis. When followed both to four cell stage or to blastocyst, a significant embryo toxic effect was seen, with progression to blastocyst stage being about one-third of normal.

Finally, work by Suginame[186-187] lead to identification of a factor which inhibits ovum capture in an in vitro hamster system. This substance was identified in cell-free PF in patients with endometriosis.

In summary:

- Peritoneal fluid volume normally increases during the follicular phase and into the secretory phase.

- There is a suggestion that volumes of PF in patients with endometriosis may be modestly increased, but except for one study, this appears to be of little clinical importance and correlates poorly with infertility.

- Macrophage activation appears to be increased with endometriosis.

- There is no consensus on behavior of prostanoids and PF with endometriosis. Also unknown is the answer to the question of whether these compounds are markers or actually causal agents in reduced fertility. They may be in response to inflammation alone, without any inherent anti-fertility effect.

- The cytotoxic effects of macrophage activation directed towards sperm and embryo development seem to be a more attractive answer to the riddle of the relationship between PF and its contents and endometriosis-induced infertility. Whether IL-1 is **the** substance is conjectural.

Notes

#17 IMMUNOLOGIC FACTORS

It is tempting to impugn immunologic mechanisms gone awry as an etiology for infertility found in association with endometriosis. As with other factors studied, such as the prostanoids, results often fail to show a consensus, and the all important sequence of causality remains unclear. Some of this material was mentioned in the preceding section on peritoneal fluid factors.

Endometriosis might result from an inheritable immunodeficiency state, or, conversely might arise from formation of autoantibodies on a humoral or cellular basis (or both). Briefly, the humoral system involves initial sensitization by an antigen followed by antibody formation by specific clones of cells, with only the antibody specific to that clone. Immunoglobulins A, D, E, G and M may result. The full antibody response usually involves complement fixation, cytolysis and phagocytosis. Cell-medicated immunologic reactions stem from lymphoid tissue (T cells usually) in a classic delayed hypersensitivity reaction.

- Initial studies by Weed and Arquembourg[188] showed complement C_3 in the endometrium of patients with endometriosis but not in controls. This could not be confirmed by Bartosik[189] et al who found C_3 or C_4 in 75% of controls. In fact, levels were negatively correlated with the stage of endometriosis.

- Numerous studies fail to reach a consensus on immunoglobulin levels in the endometrium as a marker or etiologic factor in infertility and/or abortion in patients with endometriosis[189-194].

- Similarly, measurement of serum complement in patients with endometriosis gave conflicting results[188,195-196].

17.

Anti Endometrial Antibodies

While serum and PF measurement of immunoglobulins and complement fractions is nonspecific, isolation and quantitation of antibodies against the endometrium is certainly site specific and could explain both infertility and abortion associated with endometriosis.

- Mathur et al[192] found hemagglutinating autoantibodies in the serum of 11 of 13 patients with endometriosis. Antibodies against ovary, granulosa cells and theca cells were present often. Seven of 13 had antibodies in cervical secretions. All 13 were positive for antibodies against endometrium from controls. IgG and IgA were more often present than IgM. Still, the question of cause and effect can be raised, i.e., does endometriosis elicit the antibody response or does altered immunity lead to endometriosis?

- Badawy et al[195] used endometrial homogenates to demonstrate serum antibodies in patients with endometriosis; controls were negative.

- Wild and Shivers[197] found antiendometrial antibodies in 28 of 34 patients with laparoscopically proven endometriosis using immunofluorescent methods.

- Only two of 38 controls were positive. For the endometriosis patients there were 21% false negatives and 10% false positives.

- Similar results were achieved by Kriener et al[198] who found IgG antibodies against the endometrium in 16 of 18 patients with laparoscopically documented endometriosis. In 24 without that diagnosis at surgery, antibody testing was positive in nine, but eight of those had evidence of chronic PID. Testing was performed by immunofluoroescence on endometrial biopsies.

- Subsequent work by Mathur's group[199] used Western blot analysis to detect both humoral and local auto-immune activity against antigens of 26 and 34 kilodaltan (kd).

- Kennedy et al[200] used an enzyme-linked immunosorbent assay (ELISA) to demonstrate a reduction in anti endometrial antibody titer following nafarelin therapy but not with danazol treatment . This was surprising given the immunoactive nature of danazol therapy and results of previous studies.[201]

- Badawy et al[202] demonstrated antiendometrial antibodies by passive hemagglutination in 88% of patients with endometriosis, with serum and PF titers higher than controls.

- All of the studies agree that there was no correlation between the stage of the disease and antibody titers. In fact, there was a trend towards higher titers with lesser stages of endometriosis.

- Kennedy et al[203] also demonstrated higher titers of cardiolipin antibodies in endometriosis patients versus controls, but levels were lower than patients with documented systemic lupus erythematosus (SLE).

- Gleicher et al[204] reported 29% of endometriosis patients testing positive for antinuclear antibody and 45% with lupus anticoagulant. In 31 patients, 65% had at least one IgG autoantibody. IgM autoantibodies were seen in 45%.

Again, we find smoke but no fire. That endometriosis is associated with alterations in immune homeostasis is undeniable; endometrium or endometrial implants could serve as the putative antigen. But is the implant the provacateur or does an autoimmune process somehow foster development of ectopic endometrium?

#18 ABORTION

Does the presence of endometriosis lead to an increased risk of abortion? This disarmingly straight-forward question has sponsored yet another debate in the literature diverted to the study of endometriosis. Some authors have examined the issue in patients who have conceived **after** diagnosis, while others have studied the outcome of the last pregnancy **preceding** diagnosis. This technique introduces recall bias as a retrospective analysis. Moreover, an adverse fertility factor might progress in severity from causing abortion to later causing infertility. Certainly, a selection bias also must be considered: namely, that women with an abortion history with or without symptoms of endometriosis are more likely to consult a fertility specialist for management.

This leads yet to another bias. Patients under active management have diagnostic tests for pregnancy–hCG determinations and ultrasonography–earlier and more often than those who serve as controls. And what about the controls, so-called normal patients in some studies and other infertile non-endometriotic patients in others. As a very basic issue, what is the background first trimester abortion rate? Obviously this depends, in great part, on the population chosen for study, and how early pregnancy tests are obtained.

Table 8[205-208] shows results of three investigations using luteal phase hCG levels for early diagnosis of pregnancy. In "normal" populations, a biochemical pregnancy rate of 31% per cycle was observed. Clinical pregnancy resulted in 20%. Overall 42% of the total pregnancies were lost.

With all of these objections, there are good data existant for pregnancy wastage. Table 9 taken from an excellent review by Hornstein[209], demonstrates remarkable consistency in large groups, with spontaneous abortion in 12.6% to 14.7%. The bias here is that patients were followed **after** obstetrical registration, so that there is a variation of entry relative to the last menses with some women aborting prior to the first scheduled obstetrical visit. The Warburton and Fraser study[210] was conducted in Montreal; the Naylor and Warburton[212] data came from the Collaborative Perinatal Study of the National Institute of Neurological Diseases and Stroke. The Shapiro et al[211] study used prospective data from the Health Insurance Plan (HIP) of greater New York while the Royal College Study[213] tracked women in England who had ceased using oral contraceptives.

The well documented effect of age was quantified by Naylor and Warburton[212] who found an abortion rate of 8.3% below 30 years of age, but 15.3% in women over 35. Shapiro et al[211] found similar figures of 7.4% and 22.4%, respectively.

One of the best "pure" prospective normal studies was done by Reed and Kelly[215] in New England and reported in 1958. An interview was conducted in 161 engaged couples in 1934.

TABLE 8
PREGNANCY WASTAGE AFTER A BIOCHEMICAL DIAGNOSIS*

		Pregnancies					
Author	No. Of Cycles	*No. Biochemical*	*Biochemical per Cycle (%)*	*No. Clinical*	*Clinical per Cycle (%)*	No. Of Losses	Total Abortion Rate
Wilcox (1988)	707	198	28	155	22	61	31%
Miller (1980)	623	152	24	102	16	64	42%
Edmonds (1982)	198	118	60	51	25	73	62%
Total	1528	468	31	308	20	198	42%

*Three major studies evaluating biochemical evidence of pregnancy in sexually active fertile women with subsequent follow-up of outcome. The total abortion rate is 42%, with a pregnancy rate per cycle of 31%.

From Grifo JA, Seifer DB: Chromosomal causes of pregnancy wastage, pps. 19-35. Infertility and Reproductive Medicine Clinics of North America, Friedman AJ (guest editor), "Recurrent Pregnancy Loss", W.B. Saunders Co., January 1991.

TABLE 9
EFFECT OF AGE ON ABORTION INCIDENCE (PERCENTAGE OF TOTAL PREGNANCIES) IN NORTH AMERICAN SERIES

Age of women Studied (yr.)	*Warburton and Fraser, Montreal,*	*Naylor, US East Coast,*	*Shapiro et al,. New York,*
20	12.2	10.0	
20-24	14.3	11.7	10.1
25-29	13.7	14.1	
30-34	15.5	14.8	13.2
35-39	18.7	16.6	
40	25.5	25.6	19.3
All ages	14.7	12.6	12.6
No. of patients:	6, 835	33, 255	11, 630

From Hornstein MD: Endometriosis and Spontaneous Abortion, pps. 175-185, Recurrent Pregnancy Loss, Infertility and Reproductive Medicine, Clinics of North America, Friedman AJ (guest editor), W.B. Saunders Company, 1991.
Adapted from Jansen[214].

TABLE 10
EFFECT OF PREVIOUS ABORTION ON ABORTION INCIDENCE

	Warburton and Fraser	Naylor and Warburton
No previous pregnancies	6.5	9.2
No previous abortions	12.3	---
One abortion	23.7	22.7
Two abortions	26.2	28.4
Three abortions	32.2	33.3

From Janson RPS: Spontaneous abortion incidence in the treatment of infertility. Am J Obstet Gynecol 143:451, 1982. Reproduced with permission of the publisher, Mosby-Year Book Inc.

Twenty years later 154 had proven to be fertile (another interesting statistic!). Of first pregnancies 11% aborted spontaneously; of 488 total pregnancies, 17% aborted spontaneously. These data are consistent with the Royal College study which, admittantly, dealt with a defined segment of the population who stopped oral contraceptives in order to conceive. Table 10 adapted from Jansen[214], shows the effect of previous abortions on subsequent pregnancy regardless of diagnosis or apparent etiology.

As early as 1942 Haydon[216] reported a series of 569 women with laparotomy findings of endometriosis. Of 262 previously pregnant (prior to surgery) 51% had experienced an abortion. Table 11 summarizes studies which

TABLE 11
SPONTANEOUS ABORTIONS PRIOR TO DIAGNOSIS OF ENDOMETRIOSIS*

Author/Year	Pregnancies	Abortion	Percent (%)
Haydon[216] 1942	262	134	51
Naples[224] 1981	37	17	46
Olive[225] 1982	158	70	44
Malinak[217] 1985	277	92	40
Groll[218] 1984	27	14	52
Metzger[219] 1986	65	41	63
FitzSimmons[220] 1987	64	29	45
Pittaway[221] 1988	157	60	38
TOTAL	1047	454	44

* Adapted from Malinak and Wheeler[219]
Data have been recalculated in some cases to reflect abortion percent by pregnancy rather than by individual patient. Ectopic pregnancies and elective terminations have been eliminated as well where data was available.

addressed the issue of abortion occurring **before** a diagnosis of endometriosis was made.

- Hahn et al[222] used a rabbit model to demonstrate endometriosis-associated reduction in fetuses continuing to develop between days 8-14 after ovulation. Moreover peritoneal fluid from these animals transferred to controls one day before artificial insemination caused a decrease in fetal implantation dropping from 82% in controls to 40%. No difference in PF

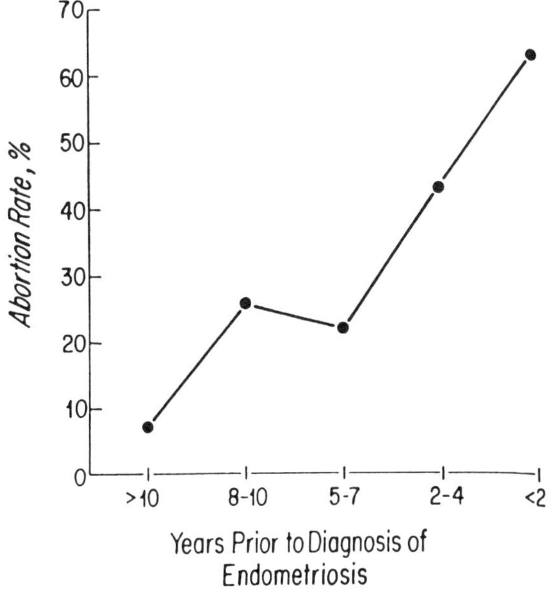

Fig. 21. Temporal relationship between diagnosis of endometriosis and abortion rate. From Naples JD, Batt RE, Sadigh H: Spontaneous abortion rate in patients with endometriosis. Obstet Gynecol 517:509, 1981. Reproduced with permission of the publisher, Elsevier Science Publishing Co., Inc.

concentration of E_2, P, or $PGF_{2\alpha}$ could be demonstrated but the adverse effect on nidation was clear.

- Rock et al[223] demonstrated a reduction of abortion from 49% to 20% in patents with endometriosis before and after surgical treatment, respectively.

- Jansen[214] demonstrated an abortion rate of only 9% following surgery for endometriosis.

- Similar results were found by Naples et al[224] who showed a reduction from 46% pre-surgery abortion rate to 8%. A subgroup treated expectantly or medically had an abortion rate of 26% following diagnosis. Most important was the finding that the abortion rate increased with proximity to the diagnosis of endometriosis (Figure 21).

- A good earlier paper on the subject was written by Olive et al[225].

- Malinak and Wheeler[217] reduced the pre-operative abortion rate from 40% by pregnancy (37% by patient) to 9% after conservative surgery based on 68 post-operative pregnancies in 63 patients.

- Groll's report[218] epitomizes the difficulty of this type of study in that, like other publications, there was no control group. But picking a true control group matched for age, and all other factors except for absence of endometriosis is almost impossible.

- To overcome this problem Metzger et al[219] compared abortion rates in patients with endometriosis managed by surgical resection or by expectant management (actually some of the latter group had monthly hydrotubations for fimbrial agglutination). Obviously patients in the advanced stages all had surgery. Table 12 shows the results of the study. Note the high abortion rate prediagnosis. No statistical

TABLE 12
PREGNANCY OUTCOME AFTER DIAGNOSIS AND SURGICAL TREATMENT OF ENDOMETRIOSIS

	No. of pregnancies	No. of SABs[a]	SAB rate
Mild			
Prediagnosis	26	11	47.8
Expectant management	18	3	16.7
Surgical excision	5	0	0.0
Moderate			
Prediagnosis	22	18	85.7
Expectant management	14	3	21.4
Surgical excision	16	0	0.0
Severe			
Prediagnosis	17	12	70.6
Expectant management	0	0	0.0
Surgical excision	11	0	0.0
Overall			
Prediagnosis	65	41	63.1
Expectant management	32	6	18.7
Surgical excision	32	0	0.0

[a]SAB, spontaneous abortion

From Metzger DA, Olive DL, Stohs GF, Franklin RR. Association of endometriosis and spontaneous abortion: effect of control group selection. Fertil Steril 45:20, 1986. Reproduced with permission of the publisher, The American Fertility Society.

difference in abortion rate was found between surgery and expectant management for mild and/or moderate disease. The authors mention recall bias and lack of tissue confirmation as factors possibly leading to a spurious high pre-diagnostic abortion rate. Second, the population was self-selected for reproductive failure. Infertile women as a group tend to have higher abortion rates regardless of the specific diagnosis. Third, the high "spontaneous cure" rate even after three abortions must be considered in all of these studies.

- FitzSimmons et al[220] approached the problem from a different angle. Women with secondary infertility having laparoscopy were divided according to absence or presence of endometriosis. The pre-diagnostic abortion rate for the endometriotic patients was 45% versus 34% (no statistical difference) for the others, confirming a generalized tendency in the infertile population toward previous reproductive failure, but not supporting a special role for endometriosis.

- Pittaway et al[221] also concluded that high spontaneous abortion rates were seen generally in patients with secondary infertility but not specifically for endometriosis.

- The literature does agree that the abortion rate prior to diagnosis of endometriosis is highest as a factor of proximity and time, but this is true as well for diagnoses of leiomyoma (as expected) and for tubal infertility as well (perhaps because of the inflammatory state as with endometriosis?).

Summary

- Studies over the last 50 years have suggested a high rate of abortion for endometriotic patients prior to diagnosis with a marked decline after surgical treatment.

- This finding may be a general one for infertile patients and not specific for endometriosis.

- All forms of statistical bias creep into these analyses, obfuscating a clear interpretation of both retrospective and prospective data.

- Since patients today are becoming increasingly more resistant to expectant management, this question is unlikely to be answered to everyone's satisfaction.

#19 THE NO TREATMENT OPTION

One of the earlier (and best) essays on treatment of endometriosis tempered by judgment was the study of Garcia and David[114] published in 1977. In an 11 year retrospective study 119 patients were studied. After laparoscopy for diagnosis (not therapy) 17 patients were found to have minimal endometriosis. Mean age in this group was 29.1 and mean duration of infertility was 3.3 years. Pregnancy occurred in 11 (65%) in this non-surgically, non-hormonally treated group within two years of laparoscopy. Eighty-six patients (all but two with moderate or severe disease) were offered conservative laparotomy, and 71 accepted surgery. Twenty-three became pregnant (32%) while only one of the 15 refusing surgery conceived. If ten patients with husbands having an adverse seminal pattern are eliminated from the surgical group, the pregnancy rate was 38%. The mean interval from surgery to pregnancy was 7.5 months (1-29). At the time, therapeutic nihilism for patients with minimal endometriosis was not fashionable, and the report engendered lively discussion. Results of "expectant management", also known as "skillful neglect" prior to the rise of litigious actions, can be assessed only with proper statistical methods. To correct for different durations of follow-up, life-table analysis has become popular. While this technique has many pluses, selection bias is still a problem. Life-table analysis can calculate the probability of pregnancy at any time during follow-up while correcting for variable duration of observation.

These cumulative pregnancy rates, however, along with calculation of fecundity rates (pregnancy per month) are based on two invalid assumptions. The first is that given time, all patients will conceive. The second is that the conception rate is constant over the interval studied; anyone who has treated infertile patients knows that this is not so. Sophisticated computer programs have allowed for corrections to be made for these factors.

- Schenken and Malinak[226] examined results of expectant management versus conservative laparotomy in mild endometriosis following a diagnostic laparoscopy. Of 16 patients with mild endometriosis and no other adverse factors, pregnancy occurred in 12 (75%) who were managed passively within an average interval of 5 months versus conception in 21 or 29 (72%) in those managed by laparotomy with an average interval of four months.

- Seibel's group[227-228] reported on a randomly selected cohort of women with minimal endometriosis assigned to six months of danazol or no treatment following diagnostic laparoscopy. Life-table analysis at 12 months after danazol cessation or laparoscopy, respectively, showed a pregnancy rate of 37% for the drug treated group versus 57% for those untreated.

- Portuondo et al[229] studied 31 couples in which the woman had laparoscopic proven but not treated endometriosis. Ten patients had donor insemination (AID/TDI) because of azoospermia. By 18 months those ten had achieved a 90% pregnancy rate. More meaningful is the fact that nine patients conceived in a total of 34 cycles of AID/TDI (mean 3.5 per patient). The remaining 21 patients had a 48% pregnancy rate by 18 months. No patient in the series conceived in the interval from 18 months to 36 months. Mean interval to pregnancy was five months for inseminated patients.

- But Jansen[230] used a group of patients receiving AID/TDI to document reduced fecundity arising from endometriosis. Laparoscopy was carried out **routinely prior** to initiation of AID/TDI. Ninety-one patients had no abnormalities in the total work-up, while seven had only minimal untreated endometriosis. Figure 22 shows a life-table demonstration of the effect of endometriosis on fecundity (0.12 for normals versus 0.036 for endometriotic women receiving frozen-thawed sperm).

- Rodriguez-Escudero[231] also studied 61 cases of minimal endometriosis managed expectantly with a subgroup of 21 requiring AID/TDI. Average duration of infertility was 4.1 years for women having AID/TDI. Expectant management led to pregnancy in 48% by 12 months in those with seminally normal husbands. In conjunction with AID/TDI, pregnancy occurred in 81% by 12 months. Monthly fecundity was 0.201 for

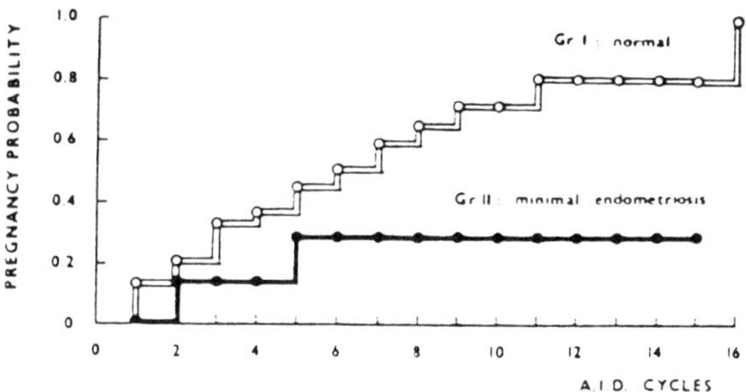

Fig. 22. Probability of pregnancy in women with endometriosis having donor insemination versus normal controls.
From Jansen RPS. Minimal endometriosis and reduced fecundability: prospective evidence from an artificial insemination by donor program. Fertil Steril 46:142, 1986. Reproduced with permission of the publisher, The American Fertility Society.

inseminated patients and 0.06 for the others. It is difficult to reach conclusions from these data. Clearly patients treated with AID/TDI who had minimal endometriosis had normal fecundity; the others, exposed to presumably normal semen did not. Should insemination be part of the empiric approach to treatment of endometriosis?

- Kable and Yussman[232] reported a series of patients in whom the pregnancy rate in those refusing therapy was 52% (9/17) with four patients of nine (44%) conceiving with mild disease, 60% (3/5) conceiving with moderate disease, and two of three (66%) who became pregnant without therapy in spite of severe endometriosis.

TABLE 13
CONCEPTION RATES IN PATIENTS WITH NO OTHER IDENTIFIABLE INFERTILITY FACTORS BY DEGREE OF ENDOMETRIOSIS

	n	Follow-up	Pregnancies	Pregnancy rate	MFR	MFR 95% confidence limits
		mos		%	%	
Mild endometriosis						
Expectant management	14	104	9	64.3	8.7	3.0 - 14.3
+ Hydrotubations	6	33	5	83.3	15.2	1.9 - 28.4
– Hydrotubations	8	71	4	50.0	5.6	0.1 - 11.2
Moderate endometriosis						
Expectant management	40	310	10	25.0	3.2	1.2 - 5.2
+Hydrotubations	9	76	3	33.3	3.9	0 - 8.4
–Hydrotubations	31	234	7	22.6	3.0	0.8 - 5.2
Severe endometriosis						
Expectant management	16	127	0	0	0	–
+ Hydrotubations	1	6	0	0	0	–
– Hydrotubations	15	121	0	0	0	–

From Olive DL, Strohs GF, Metzger DA, Franklin RR: Expectant management and hydrotubations in the treatment of endometriosis-associated infertility. Fertil Steril 44:39, 1985. Reproduced with permission of the publisher, The American Fertility Society.

- Olive et al[233] studied 70 patients managed expectantly in whom the infertility investigation had shown endometriosis as the only adverse findings. Table 13 is taken from their report. Follow-up was as long as 25 months. Even in the moderate group, both monthly fecundity rate and pregnancy rate was impressive. No pregnancies occurred in the severe group. Patients demonstrating fimbrial agglutination at laparoscopy had hydrotubation as a monthly therapy and although there is a trend toward higher fecundity, statistical significance was not reached.

- In a prospective, but not randomized study, Hull et al[234] compared no treatment, danazol for six months, or oral MPA for 90 days. For stages AFS I and II, and with follow-up of at least 18 months, 55% of controls had conceived versus 46% of the danazol patients and 71% of MPA users. No differences by stage was demonstrated. Abortion rates were 14%, 11% and 6% respectively.

- Paulson et al[235] concluded, in a recent study, that CO_2 laser use at laparoscopy was indeed better than expectant management, two modalities of pharmacologic therapy and equal to laparotomy (Table 14). Today, getting patients to enter a non-treatment arm of a multicentric study, especially when laparoscopy is involved is almost impossible. Rather, patients calling the office to make an appointment for consultation want assurance that the doctor is laser qualified.

TABLE 14
RESULTS OF TREATING ENDOMETRIOSIS WITH NO OTHER PREDISPOSING FERTILITY FACTORS

Stage		No. of patients	No. of pregnancies	% pregnant
I	Expectant	28	16	57
	Medical	95	51	54
	Danazol	77	40	52
	Medroxyprogesterone acetate	18	11	57
	Laparoscopy (cautery)	19	9	47
	Laser laparoscopy	181	147	81
	Laparotomy	116	97	84
II	Medical	59	23	39
	Danazol	52	20	38
	Medroxyprogesterone acetate	7	3	43
	Laser laparoscopy	115	80	70
	Laparotomy	62	46	74

From Paulson JD, Asmar P, Saffan DS: Mild and moderate endometriosis. Comparison of treatment modalities for infertile couples. J Reprod Med 36:151, 1991. Reproduced with permission from the Journal of Reproductive Medicine.

TABLE 15
EXPECTANT MANAGEMENT OF MINIMAL TO MILD ENDOMETRIOSIS IN OTHERWISE NORMAL WOMEN: CONCEPTION RATES

Author	Number	Follow-up Mos.	Pregnancy Rate-%	Fecundity (Monthly)
Garcia[124]	17	24	65	
Schenken[226]	16	12	75	
Bayer[228]	36	12	57	
Portuondo[229]	21	36	48	0.08 for 31
	10 (AID)	36	90	pts at 18 mos
Rodriguez-	40	12	48	0.06
Escudero[231]	21 (AID)	12	81	0.20
Olive[233]	14	25	64	0.09
Hull[234]	56	30	55	
Paulson[235]	28	36	57	

SUMMARY

Table 15 summarizes the literature on expectant management of minimal to mild endometriosis. Inspection causes one to conclude that this philosophy of patient care is reasonable. Getting patients to accept it is another matter. Delay of medical treatment has to commend it a substantial saving on pharmacologic expenses, absence of drug side-effects, and avoidance of a six month interval during which conception cannot occur.

In addition, even non-operative consultation in which no medication is prescribed may have considerable therapeutic benefit as a consequence of discussion of coital timing and techniques, and by persuasion to change life styles and habits impacting negatively on fertility.

Since the diagnosis is usually made at the time of laparoscopy, the study of Paulson et al[235] is important since conception rates with laser therapy were no worse (actually better) than when diagnostic laparoscopy only was performed. Most of the studies reported here were of women infertile for two years or more, and who had a thorough evaluation.

Actually, laparoscopy itself may be therapeutic for patients who are infertile with or without endometriosis. Tubal lavage may improve tubal function by removing inspissated mucus and other soft debris. Olive et al[233] noted a trend toward increased pregnancy rate with hydrotubation.

In an unrelated study we found that when gamete intrafallopian transfer (GIFT) was performed in patients with endometriosis, active laser management produced a trend towards pregnancy rates higher than when electrosurgery or no active treatment of the endometriosis was performed.[236]

My personal approach has been to use the laser (I don't think it matters which type) for eradication of endometriosis found at laparoscopy. If pregnancy does not occur in a reasonable interval of time dependent on the age of woman, duration of infertility and other associated factors, other therapies can be initiated. If all of the lesions cannot be ablated, or if the symptoms worsen during the observation interval, usually 6-12 months, pharmacologic therapy can be given.

Notes

#20 MEDICAL THERAPY

DANAZOL

Danazol has been the gold standard of medical treatment for endometriosis for almost two decades, and continues to be widely employed for this indication. Therefore, we shall spend some time on basic pharmacology, clinical results and side effects.

STRUCTURE:

Danazol has the cyclopentanophenanthrene steroid configuration with an ethinyl group at the 17-alpha position functioning as an alkyl radical. An isoxazol ring is attached to the A-ring (Figure 23).

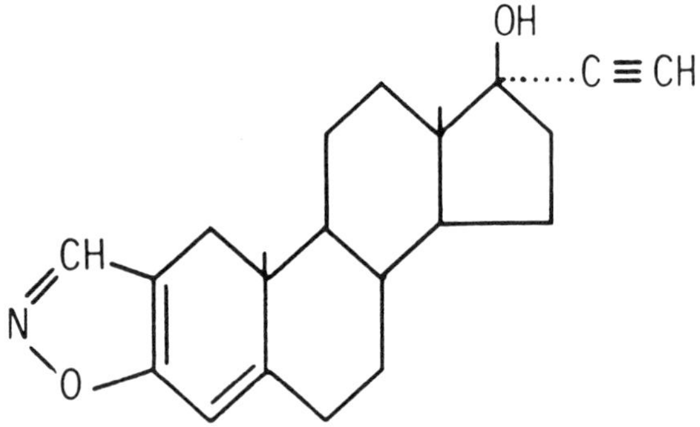

OH

C ≡ CH

CH

N

O

Fig. 23. Structural formula of danazol.

Much is held in common with the structure of testosterone, and indeed, danazol is properly characterized chemically as an isoxazol derivative of 17-alpha-ethinyltestosterone (ethisterone).

An excellent early review of danazol was published by Dmowski in 1979[237]. He summarized metabolic studies such as that performed by Davison et al [238] which demonstrated serum levels of 80ng/mL two hours after administration of a single 400mg oral dose. Observed serum half-life was 4.5 hours. Excretion studies in monkeys showed equal fecal and urinary components. Many metabolites, some with androgenic properties, have been described. One person who has been involved with danazol both in the laboratory and clinically from the outset is Robert L. Barbieri. A recent review by him[239] summarizes its pharmacology, and is heartily recommended for those wanting a more detailed account than the one presented here. Barbieri and colleagues demonstrated danazol inhibition on the following enzyme systems:

- cholesterol side-chain cleavage systems
- 3-beta-hydroxysteroid dehydrogenase
- 17-alpha-hydroxylase, 17, 20-lyase
- 17-ketosteroid oxidoreductase
- 11-beta-hydroxylase
- 21-hydroxylase
- aromatase

In many cases the danazol-induced inhibition was shown to be a result of an effect on cytochrome 450, which is an enzyme system for terminal electron transfer. The same laboratory group also demonstrated direct binding of danazol to:

- rat prostate androgen receptor
- rat uterus progesterone receptor
- rat uterus estrogen receptor (poorly)
- rat liver glucocorticoid receptor

EFFECT ON STEROID BINDING PROTEINS-TESTOSTERONE CHANGES

Danazol binds to sex hormone binding globulin (SHBG) and to corticosteroid binding globulin (CBG). Data from Nilsson et al [240-241] on the effect of danazol on testosterone binding appears in tabular form (Table 16).

Thus, the androgen effect of danazol is a consequence not only of its own inherent molecular structure, but occurs also as a result of displacement of testosterone from SHBG. Moreover, the albumin portion is less tightly bound than with SHBG. Carlstrom et al[242] showed that danazol decreases serum DHEA and DHEA-S primarily as an ovarian rather than an adrenal effect. Moreover, renal and hepatic metabolic changes in turnover were thought to play a major role in the alterations found.

TABLE 16
TESTOSTERONE BINDING IN SERUM*

	Controls %	with Danazol %
SHBG Bound	60	18
Albumin Bound	39	80
Free	1	2

*Data from Nilsson et al[240-241]

DANAZOL AND OVARIAN STEROID PRODUCTION

Steingold et al[243] found that FSH levels were not altered in patients taking danazol, but they did find elevated LH levels. Stimulation with exogenous gonadotropins documented that in danazol patients estradiol levels were about 50% less than when controls were similarly stimulated. Pregnenolone was increased; 17-hydroxypregnenolone was decreased. This finding is best explained by inhibition of 17-alpha-hydroxylase. Thus, an apparent direct effect by danazol on the ovary rather than on pituitary gonadotropes best explains these findings.

Tsang et al[244] found danazol to inhibit progesterone (P) secretion in cultures of granulosa cells and separately in thecal cell cultures even when LH was used as a stimulus. Slightly different results were noted by Olsson et al[245]. Granulosa cells in culture exposed to danazol had variable P secretion but P production stimulated by hCG was dose dependently, reversibly, decreased by addition of danazol. Using testosterone (T) as a precursor, E_2 production by the ovary also decreased under similar clinical conditions. Asch et al[246] studied monkeys given danazol in the luteal phase and demonstrated decreased P production after hCG stimulation. Henderson and Tsang[247] attributed these findings to an effect on mitochondrial cytochrome P-450. Rabe et al[248] also demonstrated an adverse effect of danazol on placental P production. In clinical use, serum E_2 levels are usually those of early follicular phase (70-140 pmol/l).

DANAZOL AND ADRENAL STEROIDOGENESIS

Stillman et al[249] showed changes in steroid patterns following ACTH stimulation in patients taking danazol that support the laboratory finding of inhibition of adrenal 3-beta-ol-hydroxysteroid dehydrogenase Δ5-Δ4 isomerase and 11-beta-hydroxylase. It is important to note that these findings are with ACTH stimulation; no cases of overt adrenal insufficiency in normal patients have arisen from use of danazol in the usually prescribed doses even over a 6-9 month interval.

DANAZOL AND HEPATIC METABOLISM

Holt and Keller[250] studied serum enzyme changes following use of danazol, at an 800mg daily dose. During a study period of up to five months using a full daily dose, significant increases in serum creatine phosphokinase, lactate dehydrogenase, and serum glutamic pyruvic transaminase were seen. Alkaline phosphatase was unchanged. These alterations resolved post-treatment. Other authors[251-253] have reported elevated enzymes on a sporadic basis in patients taking danazol. These changes are usually of no clinical importance and occur because of danazol's 17 alpha-alkylated 19-substituted structure. Patients susceptible to these changes, as with some of the 19-nor progestins, may experience a chemical hepatitis sufficient to cause the drug to be halted.

Of more recent interest, and potentially more important to the general population using danazol in repeated courses, are the changes in lipoprotein patterns.

- Allen and Frazer[254] in 1981 noted decreases in high density lipoprotein (HDL) cholesterol associated with danazol use (an effect probably mediated by T changes as well). They warned about possible atheromatous sequelae as a consequence of repeated danazol ingestion in patients who already had low HDL levels.

- Luciano et al[255] found similar results with HDL dropping by 40% within four weeks after therapy was begun.

- The national multicentric nafarelin-danazol study[107] reached similar conclusions, and also found an elevation of low density lipoprotein (LDL) cholesterol.

- Fahraeus et al[256] found not only reductions of HDL fractions with danazol use, but noted as well an LDL rise of 14%. These changes reversed within 8 weeks after the danazol was halted.

The long term effects of danazol on atherogenesis have not been elucidated past the point of these reversible lipoprotein changes. Nevertheless good clinical judgement would preclude use of this agent in patients with a family history of early adverse cardiovascular events, or in those who already have unfavorable lipoprotein profiles.

Barbieri[239] has cataloged other liver enzymatic changes including:

- increased pre-albumin
- increased C-1-esterace inhibitor
- increased haptoglobin
- increased transferrin
- increased antithrombin III
- increased prothrombin and plasminogen
- decreased SHBG
- decreased thyroid binding globulin (TBG)

DANAZOL AND GONADOTROPINS

Although the early workers postulated an antigonadotropic action to explain the clinical findings of amenorrhea and regression of endometriotic lesions seen with danazol use, this explanation has fallen by the wayside.

- In a review, Barbieri and Ryan[257] concluded that danazol actually caused an increase in basal LH and no change in FSH basal levels, although by inhibition of follicular development mid-cycle surges of both these gonadotropins were abolished. Serum prolactin was found to actually decrease[258] with danazol use, which may explain, in part, the clinical efficacy of the drug in treating fibrocystic breast disease and mastodynia with the androgenic changes and hypoestrogenemia as other components. Thyroid stimulating hormone (TSH), growth hormone (GH) and ACTH are unaffected.[239]

- Fraser et al[259] conducted GnRH stimulation studies in patients taking danazol and concluded that the drug did not impair hypothalamic or pituitary responsiveness.

- Luciano et al[260] actually noted increased responsiveness of FSH and LH release following GnRH stimulation in women taking danazol.
- Braun et al[261] and Bevan[262] also concluded that danazol did not function as a gonadotropin inhibitor.

- Dmowski et al[263] found that danazol caused a decrease in frequency of spontaneous LH pulses, but that pulse amplitude and increment increased. FSH showed no change.

DANAZOL AND THE ENDOMETRIUM

If danazol causes endometriotic lesions to regress, and to become, in part, metabolically less active, then the endometrium itself should assume a basal-like state. This is usually true, and biopsies are expected to show a basal or early follicular type picture. But as Barbieri points out[239], laboratory studies show a mixed pattern of agonist-antagonist on P receptor systems. Thus, biopsy of the endometrium, particularly in women who continue to menstruate while on therapy, occasionally may show a pseudosecretory pattern.

IMMUNOSUPPRESSIVE EFFECTS OF DANAZOL

- Hill et al[264] showed that lymphocyte proliferation in cultures activated by T-cell mitogens was inhibited in the presence of 10^{-6} M danazol. Comparable inhibition was reached with dexamethasone at 10^{-8}M. The concentration of danazol was that achieved with a daily oral dose of 600 mg.

- Mori et al[265] demonstrated that danazol suppresses production of interleukin-1B and tumor necrosis factor by human monocytes.

- Other clinical uses of danazol, treatment of immune thrombocytopenic purpura as an example,[266] clearly demonstrate an immunosuppressive effect.

- El-Roeiy et al[201] were able to show a danazol effect on autoantibodies in patients with endometriosis. Total immunoglobulin concentrations (IgG, IgA, IgM) were reduced with danazol, but not with use of a GnRH analog. These findings contradict those of Kennedy et al[200]

CLINICALLY ENCOUNTERED SIDE EFFECTS ASSOCIATED WITH USE OF DANAZOL

Figure 24 details side-effects of danazol at 800mg daily compared with nafarelin, 400ug daily, with data taken from a multicentric study.[267] The complaints are expected, in large part, as a consequence of increased free T, in addition to the androgenicity of danazol itself, coupled with the relative steady state of hypoestrogenism.

Other side effects, some expected, some not, have been reported, usually on a single case report basis, or in clusters.

- Goulbourne and MacLeod[268] called attention to the interaction between danazol and warfarin. With the danazol reducing production of vitamin K-dependent clotting factors in the liver, anticoagulants may be potentiated.

- Mercaitis et al[269] documented a non-reversible reduction in vocal pitch present 12 months after danazol had been discontinued. This drug is therefore, in my opinion, contraindicated for those who are either professional vocalists or serious singers.

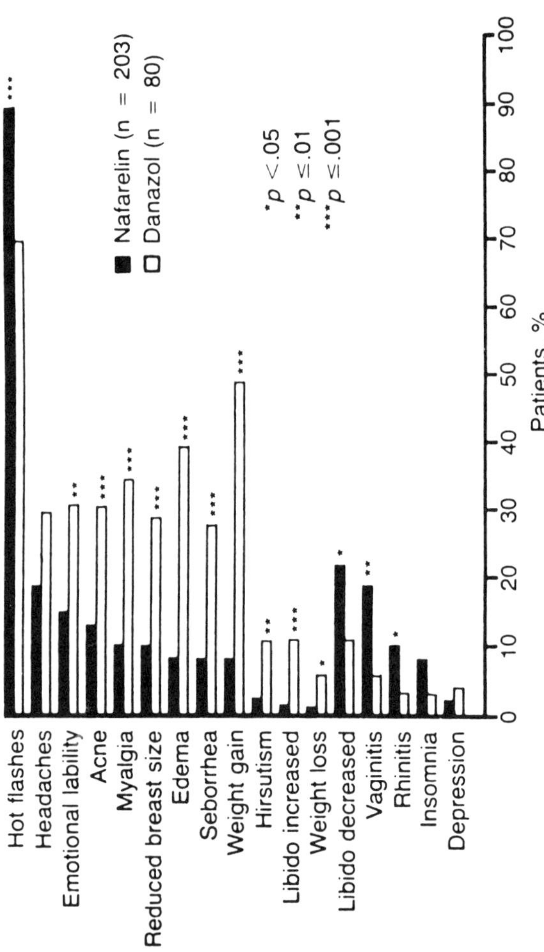

Fig. 24. Clinical side effects encountered with use of danazol versus nafarelin for therapy of endometriosis.

From Henzl MR, Kwei L: Efficacy and safety of nafarelin in the treatment of endometriosis. Am J Obstet Gynecol 162:570, 1991. Reproduced with permission of the publisher, Mosby-Year Book, Inc.

- Bilateral sensorineural hearing loss associated with danazol has also been described.[270]

- Carpal tunnel syndrome has been reported as well[271], with fluid retention given as a possible etiology.

- Most important has been the adverse effect of danazol on the developing female fetus. Virilization is to be expected as the drug crosses the placenta. Duck and Katayama[272] reported a case of female pseudohermaphroditism in 1981. This was followed by other reports[273-276] in the literature.

While patients should be advised to contracept mechanically during the entire interval of danazol use, this meets with poor compliance. Rather, a negotiable compromise that is likely to succeed is to insist on mechanical contraception during the first 4-6 weeks of use, assuming a daily dose of at least 600 mg daily that is expected to block ovulation reliably.

DANAZOL TREATMENT AND SUBSEQUENT FERTILITY

Since most of the studies concerned with expectant management use danazol as the treated group for comparison, the reader is referred back to section 19 in order to avoid repetition of those data. Additional information appears in the discussion of danazol used primarily for pain control in section 13. The studies about to be cited suffer collectively from lack of control groups in many cases, weak statistical methodology and inclusion of patient-couples with additional adverse fertility findings, yet they represent the best information available.

Dmowski and Cohen in 1978[277] reported on danazol primarily used for treatment of infertility in 90 patients. A dose of 800 mg daily was employed. Amenorrhea during the 3-18 month course of therapy (average 6 months) was reached by 66%, with 28% having spotting and 3% with irregular bleeding.

- Pregnancy was achieved by 39, divided as 53% for those with mild endometriosis, 46% for moderate disease and 28% for those with severe pathology. "Correction" for other severe fertility factors such as poor seminal quality or tubal obstruction gave respective values of 83%, 73% and 38%.

- The majority of conceptions occurred within 6 months following completion of therapy.

- Nine of the pregnancies were achieved with additional therapies such as ovulation induction.

Biberoglu and Behrman278 studied the effect of danazol dosage from 100mg through 600mg daily when used for endometriosis.

- At doses of 100, 200, 400, or 600 mg daily amenorrhea was achieved by 29%, 38%, 86% and 88% of patients respectively.

- Regardless of dose used, endometriomas of the ovary >1 cm responded poorly, one of the few consistent findings in the literature.

- Pregnancy was achieved by five of eleven patients who were infertile; three were with the 600mg daily dose, one had taken 100mg daily and one was in a patient during a course of 200mg daily.

- Side-effects seemed not to be related to the daily dose.

One particularly good study was done as a six center investigation and was reported by Butler et al[279]. Following laparoscopic documentation of endometriosis 75 otherwise normal infertile patients were given danazol, usually 800mg daily for 6 months. The danazol was started three months after surgery to allow, in part, for a possible therapeutic effect of laparoscopy alone. The range of follow-up was 12-34 months, and 95% were followed for 18 months or longer.

- Pregnancy rate for mild endometriosis was 28% with a 29% first trimester abortion rate.

- Pregnancy rate ranged from 14% to 40% among the six centers demonstrating the inherent statistical weakness of individual small studies.

- Pregnancy occurred in 31% of those on 800mg daily, which was greater, but not statistically so, than the rate for those on smaller doses.

DANAZOL VERSUS GnRH ANALOGS FOR TREATMENT OF ENDOMETRIOSIS-ASSOCIATED INFERTILITY

Studies in which danazol is compared with GnRH analogs tend to have the advantage of better protocol construction as a consequence of investigators becoming more knowledgeable and sophisticated about statistical methodology. The prototype of these head-to-head studies[107] has already been discussed in the section on pain control. A subsequent publication by Henzl and Kwei[267] examined a slightly expanded data base using the same double-blind randomized protocol. Nafarelin, 400 ug daily was taken by 204 patients, 79 received 800 ug daily and 67 took danazol 600mg daily while 80 patients had 800mg of danazol daily for 6 months. Even with this excellent protocol, a problem of methodology taints the follow-up evaluation. Although active laparoscopic therapy was interdicted at the first diagnostic procedure, it was not during the second procedure following completion of 6 months of therapy. Thus, fertility rates easily might be affected by lysis of adhesions or laser therapy of residual implants following use of any of the agents. This possibility is of equal potential for all of the subgroups, but still detracts somewhat from the results.

- Figure 24 (pg. 166), depicts in graphic form the comparative side-effects of therapy. In this study it is clear that danazol has a wider and more severe range of adverse effects than nafarelin.

- Of 149 women attempting to conceive, 52% who took nafarelin, 800 ug daily, were successful by 12 months following therapy. 30% conceived with the 400 ug per day dose and 36% conceived after danazol use. These differences were not statistically significant.

There is no evidence that pregnancy rates are enhanced or adversely affected by the use of Synarel.

Fedele et al[280] studied 32 patients given 600 mg of danazol daily versus 30 patients given 1200 ug of buserelin (a GnRH analog popular in Europe) daily for 6 months. At second look laparoscopy regression of lesions was not different by drug group, and pain relief was also similar. At 18 months the cumulative pregnancy rate for buserelin patients was 48% versus 43% for the danazol group (no difference).

DANAZOL AND SURGERY FOR ENDOMETRIOSIS-ASSOCIATED INFERTILITY

This question, not surprisingly, is one with conflicting answers from the literature. Should danazol be given preoperatively to reduce the activity and size of lesions, lessening the inflammatory response in order to improve surgical planes especially for laparoscopic procedures? Or, does this therapy hide lesions by temporarily making them less visible? Does post-operative use a danazol intrude on the most fertile window of time-those six months following surgery?

Buttram has published a number of articles dealing with this question, culminating in a six year analysis of a prospective study. [281-283] He concluded that:

- Resolution of ovarian endometrioma >1cm was poor with danazol therapy.
- Fifty percent of 16 patients with minimal disease and 39% of 33 with mild disease conceived with drug therapy alone.
- Fifteen of 18 (83%) patients with mild, 18/27 (67%) with moderate and 15 of 30 (50%) patients with severe disease conceived after 6 months of 400-800mg of danazol daily followed by surgery. This was a higher pregnancy rate than treatment with drug alone.
- Of 24 patients treated for 6 months with danazol after surgery, conception occurred in 30% independent of danazol dose.
- Preoperative use was associated with reduced tissue inflammation and vascularity. Pregnancy rates were improved regardless of stage. The 800 mg daily dose seemed slightly more efficacious than the 400mg daily dose.

But Wheeler and Malinak[284], at the same institution, (Baylor College of Medicine) concluded that post-operative use of danazol was indeed helpful, noting a post-surgical pregnancy rate of 30% in 199 having laparotomy alone versus 79% (15/19) in those having surgery then 400mg of danazol daily for three to six months.

Guzick and Rock[285] retrospectively studied 91 patients treated with danazol for mild or moderate endometriosis versus 133 treated by conservative laparotomy for infertility. Patients had been infertile for at least one year with no other pathology found. Most, (72/91 patients) received 800mg of danazol daily for 6 months. Life-table analysis showed a virtually identical cumulative pregnancy rate - 68% surgical, 74% danazol.

Donnez et al[286] prospectively studied women with laparoscopically proven ovarian endometriosis who were treated with danazol for 6 months prior to a planned microsurgical laparotomy. Other patients received gestrinone or buserelin. By definition, these cases were in the moderate to severe category.

- Lesions were observed to decrease in size, remain the same, or actually increase with all three therapies, but buserelin was clearly superior.

- The cumulative pregnancy rate following pre-operative preparation with buserelin and then surgery was 58% at 18 months, which was superior to the comparable values for danazol and/or gestrinone.

SUMMARY

Danazol remains a first-line therapeutic agent for pharmacologic therapy of endometriosis-related infertility. The literature is not clear on its use as primary therapy or in the proper sequence when used with surgery. My own guidelines and philosophy of management follow.

- Since diagnosis is usually made at the time of laparoscopy, destruction of lesions at that time is desirous. If pregnancy has not occurred within 6-9 months, or if symptoms of endometriosis rapidly reappear, medical therapy may be initiated.

- Daily doses of 600-800mg, often on a patient weight basis, seems reasonable over a 3-6 month interval. Lesser doses are associated with more troublesome breakthrough bleeding and may be slightly less efficacious. Severe disease, only, may profit from longer duration of treatment.

- The appearance of the GnRH analogs clinically gives us a pharmacologic choice dependent more on selection of potential side effects than differences in efficacy. An asthenic patient with a family history of early osteoporosis is a much better danazol choice than an obese, hypertensive patient with adverse lipoprotein patterns and a family history of cardiovascular disease.
- If a previous laparoscopy or current pelvic examination suggests fixation of pelvic structures as a consequence of inflammatory adhesions, preoperative suppression for 3-6 months may allow for operative laparoscopy rather than laparotomy. I have seen tremendous reduction of tissue reaction with reappearance of surgical planes after such treatment.

- In my own experience, danazol is somewhat effective in shrinking the volume of endometriomas preoperatively, but less so than GnRH analogs.

GnRH ANALOG THERAPY FOR ENDOMETRIOSIS-ASSOCIATED INFERTILITY

Native GnRH is shown in Figure 25 as a decapeptide. The spacial configuration is such that amino acid bonds 5, 6 and 7 are most susceptible to pituitary endopeptidase cleavage. Carboxyamide peptidase is active at bond 9-10. Serum half-life is in the range of 2-8 minutes.

Studies indicate that amino acids 1, 6 and 10 confer structural configuration necessary for binding to pituitary receptors, but receptor activation is localized to sites 2 and 3.[287-288] Activation occurs through the mechanism of calcium entry into the cell causing exocytotic release of secretory granules containing LH or

Gonadotropin Releasing Hormone

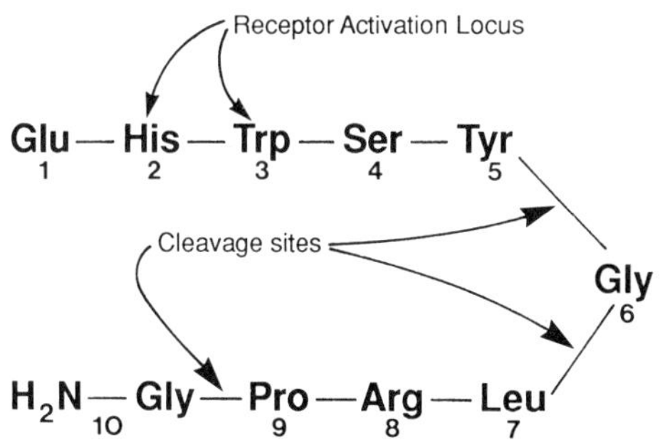

Fig. 25. Structural formula of endogenous GnRH.

FSH. Actual synthesis is stimulated by activation of protein kinase C which in turn, increases phosphorylation in the cystosol. Potency is usually gained through substitution at position 10. Substitution here also can reduce proteolysis. Changes at position six with D but not L steroisomers give agonistic properties and greatly alters half-life. Substitutions at positions 6 and 10 are often synergistic. Table 17 shows potencies relative to the naturally occurring molecule. In vivo potency may actually be different and bioassays frequently give lower values for LH than radioimmunoassay (RIA).

To summarize the brilliant work of Knobil[289], hourly pulses of native GnRH were found to restore pituitary release of FSH and LH in monkeys who had been prepared with

TABLE 17
AMINO ACID SUBSTITUTIONS AND IN VITRO POTENCIES OF SOME GnRH AGONISTS

GnRH agonist	Substitution	Potency*	Half-life Min
Buserelin	D-Ser (tBu),^{6} Pro^9	50	80
Goserelin	D-Ser (tBu), (Aza-Gly-NH$_2$)^{10}	100	360
Nafarelin	D-Nal (2)^6	200	260
Leuprolide	D-Leu^6-Pro^9	50	180
Decapeptyl	D-Trp^6	36	----
Histrelin	imbzl - D-His^6 -Pro^9	100	----

* Relative to natural GnRH

hypothalamic lesions, whereas a continuous IV infusion caused suppression following a short burst of initial stimulation. This biphasic response—with an initial short stimulatory arm and a longer inhibitory arm—has been found in normal women.[290] This phenomenon has been ascribed to two different mechanisms of action. The first is that of desensitization which uncouples the binding complex from its intracellular sequelae. The second is downregulation which denotes a lessened number of unoccupied receptor sites.

THE AGONISTS-GENERAL COMMENTS

Currently two agonists are FDA approved for clinical use in the United States, leuprolide acetate (LA, Lupron TAP/Abbott), and nafarelin acetate (NA, Synarel-Syntex). In Canada, nafarelin acetate still remains at the time of writing , the only GnRH-a which is HPB approved for treatment of endometriosis.

Nafarelin acetate (Synarel-Syntex) is clinically delivered as a metered nasal spray with the usual dose being 200 μg in one of each nostril at 12 hour intervals. Oral routes are not effective for any of the analogues because of gastrointestinal enzymatic degradation. Bioavailability of the nasally delivered drug is 2-5% of the intravenous (IV) route. A few patients may not become totally amenorrheic after two months of treatment with 400 μg of nafarelin daily. An increase to 800 μg daily given as 400 μg (1 spray into each nostril) at 12 hour intervals may be necessary in such cases. Bleeding,

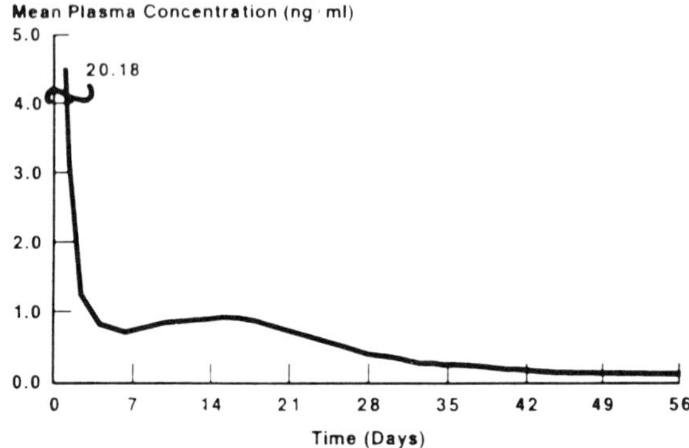

Fig. 26. Serum levels (man) of Leuprolide acetate following intramuscular 7.5 mg injection.

*Courtesy Dr. J. Miller, TAP Pharmaceuticals, N. Chicago, IL

itself, is not always a good indicator of sufficient levels of inhibition since some women bleed from a basal endometrium which is already maximally suppressed.

I shall confine my comments with respect to leuprolide acetate mainly to the depot form. That preparation has as its structure biodegradable 20 μm microspheres containing the drug. Figure 26 demonstrates initial release after a 7.5 mg injection with sustained stable levels over the next 30 days or so. Depot preparations are packaged as 7.5 mg 3.75 mg injections with no preservative so that the drug must be used within 24 hours of opening the package. Deep suppression can be accomplished with a larger dose although menses will usually return by 8 weeks after cessation. My own protocol is to give the 7.5 mg as the initial dose for a reliable quick suppression, and 3.75 mg at 30 day intervals for sustained suppression thereafter.

Cycle timing of initial administration should be considered. Suppression occurs more quickly if mid to late luteal phase is employed as the initial start, but pregnancy must first be ruled out by means of a serum beta-hCG evaluation. Conversely, initiation of therapy in the late follicular phase may result in a longer stimulation pattern with production of simple ovarian cysts which eventually regress as inhibition sets in. Most patients will suppress within five to twelve days, with that definition being serum estradiol levels of 25 pg/ml (75pmol/L) or less.

MONITORING

The best way to monitor therapy is to simply measure serum estradiol. Depending on the laboratory, any value of 25 pg/mL (75 pmol/L) or less is in the range of adequate suppression. Amenorrhea is usually reached after the next expected menses, i.e. within 6-8 weeks following initiation of therapy. We suggest a routine determination of serum E_2 about 6 weeks after therapy has been initiated (although this is not a recommendation of the manufacturer), and again only if the patient has significant breakthrough bleeding or worsening of symptoms. Serial CA 125 measurements are not very helpful in following the effect of the drug on endometriosis. After a baseline ultrasound examination has demonstrated a presumed endometrioma, a follow-up study at 3 months should show some decrease in size. If this is not the case, clinical judgment must be employed as to whether a longer interval of suppression is necessary, or whether surgery should be done at an earlier date since the lesion may not be an endometrioma at all. Women with a history of endometriosis do, in fact, get other ovarian lesions, both benign and malignant, and therefore this becomes not only theoretical, but a real problem in clinical practice. Significant change in lipoprotein pattern is not an important consideration with analog therapy. Side effects have been mentioned already in conjunction with danazol comparison and are best treated symptomatically. Vaginal lubricants may be necessary to overcome local atrophic changes. The issue of "estrogen-give back" will be discussed separately.

BONE DENSITY

The very factor that makes analog use so attractive for endometriosis therapy—the ability to achieve sustained menopausal levels of serum estrogen—also makes for the most potentially long term troubling side effect, that of accelerated osteoporotic changes. Before discussing this, it is important to note that the literature is a quagmire of opinions on this issue as a consequence of:

- Different techniques of assessment of bone mineral content.
- Description of cortical versus trabecular bone changes.

- The sites measured.
- Depth and duration of ovarian suppression.
- Calcium supplementation during analog therapy.

Routine bone density studies prior to therapy are neither recommended nor cost effective. Probably dual photon absorptiometry (DPA) is the most versatile method of measurement since it has both lower cost and lower dose of radiation than computerized tomography, and it can measure cortical as well as trabecular bone and central bone density. Dual X-ray absorptiometry (DEXA) is a newer technique which shows great promise.

Thus, some studies done with pre-therapy evaluation and then repeat examination after (usually) six months of analog therapy, show no bone loss[291-294]. Other studies[295-297] suggest a decreased density which is reversible by 6 months following cessation of drug therapy. Dawood et al[298] noted a 7% decrease in vertebral body trabecular bone density after 6 months of buserelin (intranasal) use. Six months after completion of therapy, density was still 4% less than baseline. Others,[296-297] have found similar early loss, but Matta et al[297] noted complete restoration of density after an interval following cessation of therapy. The early bone loss probably mimics the changes which occur with spontaneous menopause, namely, that bone loss is initially rapid and then tapers off with time.

The waters were further muddied with results from a study by Comite et al[299] who suggested that women with endometriosis had a bone loss reduction in association with that diagnosis prior to therapy. This was not the findings of Lane et al[300] who also conducted baseline studies.

Jacobson[301] found negligible bone loss after 6 months of nafarelin use at 200 ug per day. With 400 ug daily, loss of bone density ranged from 2% to 6% by 6 months. But patients on this dose who also received norethindrone 1.2 mg daily showed no loss. The studies of Riis et al[109] and Surrey et al[110] mentioned previously, also document the ability of norethindrone to lessen bone loss in patients receiving analog therapy without detracting from therapeutic effect. Thus, the rational for progestin "add-back" or "give-back" therapy.

Dodin et al[302] studied the effect of goserelin (Zoladex-ICI Pharma) versus danazol on bone mass. The latter had no effect on bone density, but by six months E_2 levels with danazol were 330 pmol/L versus 68.6 pmol/L for the analog. With goserelin, lumbar spine and femoral neck losses were 8.2% and 7.7% of density respectively, at six months of therapy. Six months following treatment, bone density values were still reduced for the analog patients, but not statistically so from pretreatment baseline studies. Such deep suppression with analogs may not be necessary for a therapeutic effect. Below a certain steady state E_2 level, additional regression of implants may not occur. Above a certain threshold of E_2, bone metabolism may be relatively unaffected, while endometriotic implants still atrophy. That magical level has not yet been found, but this brings us to a discussion of "give back."

ESTROGEN "GIVE-BACK"

This concept is still experimental and under current clinical evaluation. Its use is not at the present time FDA or HPB approved.

The estrogen threshold hypothesis popularized by Barbieri and Friedman, in particular, holds that there may be a differential threshold for activation of endometriotic implants which is (it is hoped) higher than the threshold below which bone resorption exceeds deposition. The progestin studies are of great clinical interest, but they do not directly address this question. A multicentric study employing pre- and post-therapy bone density evaluation as well as laparoscopy will be necessary to satisfactorily define these limits of interaction between analog therapy and estrogen replacement with respect to bone density behavior and efficacy of endometriotic therapy. Until then an oblique answer may be found in data accumulated from studies of women given estrogens following hysterectomy and ovarian removal for endometriosis. Recurrence of endometriosis following a surgically created menopause is in the neighborhood of 9%[303-305], but the proportion of women with residual implants following pelvic organ extirpation, i.e. the actual number of women at risk, is unknown. The problem is really one of interaction of two drugs on the target cells, and there will probably be a spectrum of clinical response with some patients needing deep suppression for regression of lesions, and with other patients actually requiring rather minor reductions of estrogen production in order to achieve a beneficial effect.

Clinical studies indicate a more profound suppression of estradiol levels using long-acting depot formulations compared to the nasal spray formulations. At the same time, bone mineral density appears to be reduced to a greater extent when a more profound hypoestrogenic state induced by the long-acting depot compared to the short-acting, intranasally administered preparations.

Several add-back studies are currently underway evaluating various estrogen and/or progestin regimens. Whether different dosages of add-back will be necessary depending on the agonist employed remains to be seen. The question is "since different agonists cause different levels of ovarian suppression, will different dosages of add-back therapy be necessary to overcome the hypoestrogenic effects?"

We have managed some of our patients with severe menopausal symptoms who are receiving analogue therapy (indicated for endometriosis) as follows:

- The initial dose is either 400 µg/day of Synarel intranasally or 7.5 mg LA intramuscularly. The dosage of Synarel is maintained at 400 µg daily or it may be increased to 800 μg daily if amenorrhea is not achieved after 2 months of therapy. If LA is employed, it is continued thereafter every 30 days as a 3.75 mg injection intramuscularly. Both therapies are employed for 6 months.

- We then add estrogen in the form of a 0.05mg Estraderm patch (Estraderm-CIBA) after 6 weeks of analog therapy. This usually gives estradiol levels of about 25-50 pg/mL (75-150 pmol/L) with approximately 40 pg (120 pmol/L) as the low figure for bone density neutrality.

- If this is insufficient, the 0.1mg patch is used. Estradiol measurements with commercially available kits used in conjunction with micronized estradiol given orally also measure some of the elevated estrone (E_1) which can be quite marked with this form of therapy. One could empirically use Estrace 1mg orally on a daily basis or could measure E_2 using a chromatographic method after extraction. This is logistically difficult and certainly not cost effective. Instead, the patient can be followed clinically.

- Conjugated equine estrogens have been used as menopausal estrogen replacement for years, but of course this mixture makes serum measurement of E_2 superfluous. The general feeling is that 0.3 mg daily is not sufficient to prevent bone density loss, and therefore 0.625 mg would be needed under these circumstances.

- The issue of "unopposed estrogen" even for 6 months in patients with intact uteri and with low level therapy remains to be addressed.

These protocols of add-back or give-back therapy are experimental and not approved for use by the FDA or HPB. They are evolving and the astute clinician will need to consult the journal literature for current thinking on this subject.

THE AGONISTS—EFFICACY

We already have presented data on a number of agonist-danazol studies[107, 267, 280]. Some of the nafarelin data show a trend towards better pregnancy rates with use of 800 mg daily[267] but statistical significance was not attained. Buserelin has been available in Europe for a longer duration of time than LA has been used in the United States, and consequently a number of different protocols for use have been investigated.

- Ronnberg et al[306] found a 54% pregnancy rate (7/13) between 10-17 months following use of 150 ug of buserelin sprayed in each nostril 3 times daily.

- Donnez et al[307], however, using second-look laparoscopy to assess regression, found this dose and route to be inferior to subcutaneous implants of buserelin given as 6.6mg at weeks 0,6 and 12 of a six month study.

GnRH ANTAGONISTS

Use of GnRH antagonists for endometriosis is only in the very early clinical evaluation stage, but would seem to be a more direct therapy than agonists if for no other reason than to avoid the stimulatory phase. The early antagonists caused severe histamine release reactions. Even with this problem apparently solved by clever biosynthesis and molecular manipulation, other factors must be considered. A pituitary gonadotrope occupancy of < 10% is sufficient to cause secretion[308], and GnRH is released in a pulsatile fashion. Therefore, an effective antagonist must have both high receptor affinity and extremely long duration of action. Not surprisingly, a high daily dose of antagonist is needed to block FSH/LH release in castrate animals and a high dose is also needed to block ovulation[309], since desensitization is not operative as it is with the agonist. An excellent discussion of agonist-antagonist therapy appears in a monograph by Barbieri and Friedman[310].

SUMMARY

- GnRH-a preparations used for endometriosis-related infertility give pregnancy rates as least as good as those seen with use of danazol.
- Side-effects are basically those of hypoestrogenemia rather than anabolic and androgenic in nature.
- Concomitant use of low dose estrogen or progestin supplements may ameliorate clinical side effects but this possibility requires further clinical investigation.

#21 SURGERY FOR ENDOMETRIOSIS ASSOCIATED INFERTILITY

In recent years, operative, as opposed to purely diagnostic, laparoscopy has surpassed laparotomy as the treatment of choice, where possible, for endometriosis-related infertility. After early studies suggested that results were at least as good, economic and cosmetic advantages, coupled with continued improvements in laparoscopic ancillary instrumentation drove the endoscopic route as the preferred treatment.

All but the most ardent and stubborn endoscopists would admit that the disease process in **some** patients is best approached by laparotomy, especially when the bowel is involved or when severe adhesive disease thwarts the laparoscopic approach. Therefore, we should first survey the results of conservative laparotomy for endometriosis.

Regardless of the route employed, the cornerstone of surgical philosophy has been one of debulking pathology by extirpation or destruction with energy (laser or electrosurgery). Thus, all visible implants should be treated. The laparotomists stressed meticulous reperitonealization of the pelvic surfaces, but even that sacred cow has been subject to attack, with data from various animal studies and from human experience as well. How many of us no longer reapproximate either the posterior or anterior peritoneal defect at laparotomy?

Uterine suspension has ridden the pendulum of great popularity through rejection as a routine ancillary therapeutic maneuver. Theory holds that when adhesive disease is severe, particularly posteriorly in and around the cul-de-sac, suspension, whether by creating a uterosacral ligamentous shelf or by one of a number of round ligament procedures, is helpful even as a temporary expedient.

Plication of the uterosacral ligament to prevent readherence of ovaries and tubes to mesocolon, in particular, seems to have some merit (Figure 27). Overzealous advancement can cause ureteral kinking. No prospective, randomized study with second-look laparoscopy or pregnancy as an end point has measured the value of routinely adding this step. Round ligament suspension to the fascia often is transient regardless of suture chosen because the ligament rapidly stretches while on tension. Post operative discomfort from this tension may be marked in the first few weeks. Care must be taken to avoid formation of small open spaces between the uterine fundus and surgically-created ligamentous attachment to anterior peritoneum and overlying fascia, because an internal hernia with strangulation of small intestine can occur (Figure 28). Care must be taken as well to avoid kinking of the proximal portion of the fallopian tube as the round ligament is sutured.

The hunt for an agent to prevent adhesion formation (reformation) has yet to be satisfactorily concluded. Intraperitoneal steroids

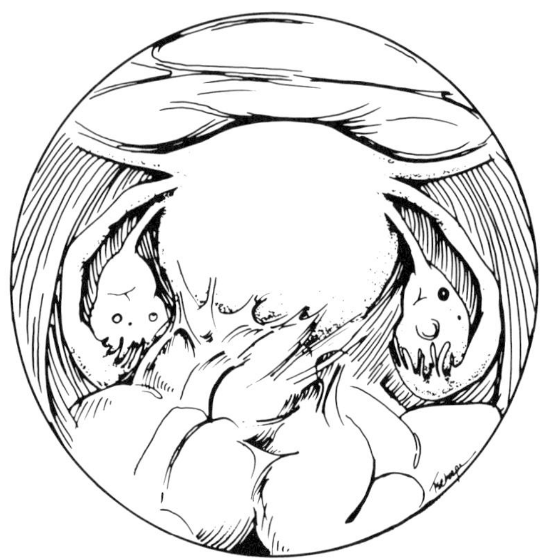

Fig. 27A. – cul-de-sac endometriosis

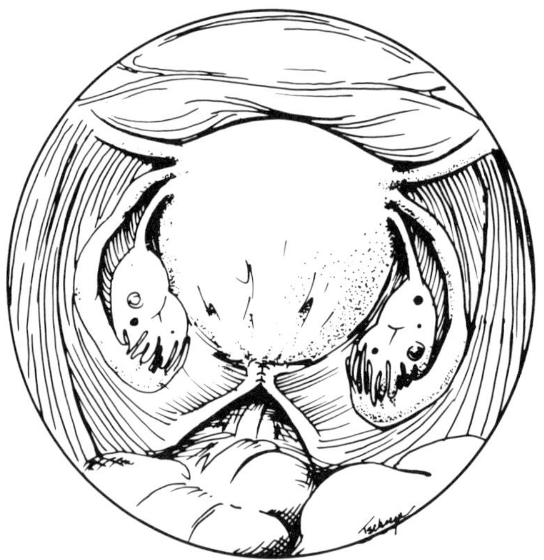

Fig. 27B. – following surgery the uterosacral ligaments have been plicated. This can be performed at laparotomy or laparoscopy.

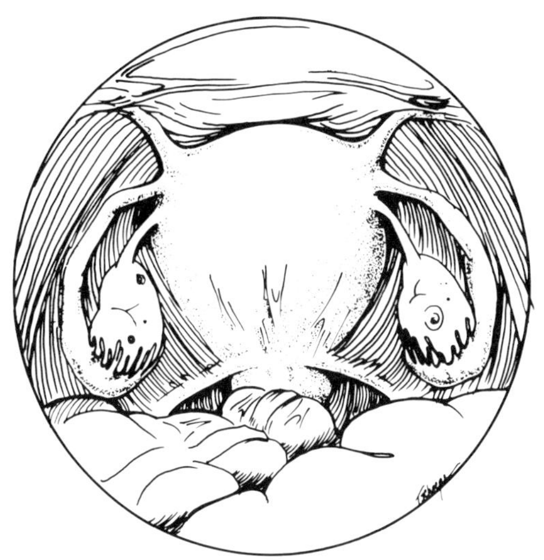

Fig. 28. Round ligament anterior uterine suspension performed laparoscopically with suture above the fascia.

were ancedotally popular but failed to stand up to scientific scrutiny in double blind studies. High molecular weight dextran has had a brief period of popularity. Various anti-inflammatory agents are in clinical trial. Mechanical barriers have been employed also, but no single agent has proven to be spectacularly effective. While the problem of adhesion prevention is not the main subject of this dissertation, it is germane to the discussion of surgical therapy for endometriosis since many women who remain infertile following surgery may actually have severe adhesions and little or no recurrent active endometriosis.

Presacral neurectomy is primarily directed toward relief of pain, and does not improve pregnancy rates as an independent procedure.[114] Evaluation of pregnancy rates following conservative laparotomy is made difficult because of variation between surgeons and techniques they employ, patient staging, associated pharmacologic therapy and unequal follow-up intervals, to name a few. In particular, many patients referred to a specialist for endometriosis surgery return to their primary doctor who may institute additional supportive therapy such as ovulation stimulation to augment fertility. Tables 18, 19 and 20 summarize literature on conservative laparotomy for endometriosis-associated infertility according to stage. In general, in spite of differences in classification schemes, a relation to stage was found.

TABLE 18
PREGNANCY AFTER CONSERVATIVE SURGERY FOR MILD ENDOMETRIOSIS

	N	% PREGNANT
Acosta et al[50] 1973	8	75
Garcia & David[114] 1977	3	67
Buttram[281] 1979	88	69
Rock et al[311] 1981	45	62
Schenken & Malinak[226] 1982	42	76
Rantala et al[312] 1983	44	59
Gordts et al[313] 1984*	20	40
Olive & Lee[314] 1986	11	46
TOTAL	261	64

*AFS Staging[50], others according to Acosta et al[51].

TABLE 19
PREGNANCY AFTER CONSERVATIVE SURGERY FOR MODERATE ENDOMETRIOSIS

	N	% PREGNANT
Acosta et al[50] 1973	60	50
Sadigh et al[315] 1977	23	74
Garcia & David[114] 1977	19	37
Schenken & Malinak[316] 1978	36	33
Buttram[281] 1979	50	56
Rock et al[311] 1981*	88	55
Rantala et al[312] 1983	39	56
Gordts et al[313] 1984*	99	42
Olive & Lee[314] 1986	43	51
TOTAL	457	50

*AFS Staging[50], others according to Acosta et al[51].

TABLE 20
PREGNANCY AFTER CONSERVATIVE SURGERY FOR SEVERE ENDOMETRIOSIS

	N	% PREGNANT
Acosta et al[50] 1973	39	33
Sadigh et al[315] 1977	42	48
Garcia & David[114] 1977	49	29
Schenken & Malinak[316] 1978	21	29
Buttram[281] 1979	68	47
Rock et al[311] 1981*	81	48
Rantala et al[312] 1983	46	39
Gordts et al[313] 1984*	57	35
Olive & Lee[314] 1986	34	29
TOTAL	439	39

AFS* Staging[50], others according to Acosta et al[51].

The Garcia and David[114] study was mentioned before as a paragon of surgical judgment in that when surgery was not advocated for minimal to mild disease, 65% conceived within two years with expectant management; but only 7% conceived who declined the suggested laparotomy. The data from the laparoscopy only patients might serve as well as a "literature" control group for expected pregnancy rate in minimal/mild disease without operative intervention. Similar results were achieved by Schenken and Malinak[226].

Buttram[281] reviewed 206 patients operated over a span of seven years. He stressed that following a conservative laparotomy 30.5% of these who conceived did so within three months, 48.8% within six months and 86.0% within 15 months.

Rock et al[311] generally agreed with the Buttram[281] observation on fertility in the immediate postoperative interval, noting that 62% of the 136 pregnancies in 115 women occurred within one year, for an overall pregnancy rate of 54%. But 31% of pregnancies occurred in the 2-3 year interval, and 7% thereafter.

They calculated fecundity rates, noting the invalid assumption of constant rate over the interval of observation. The actual fecundity rate (r) dropped from 0.03 per month in the first year to 0.005 in the sixth year post operatively. Patients with ovarian endometriomas in excess of 3 cm had poor fertility results. Duration of infertility and parity had no prognostic significance.

Rantala et al[312] conversely found duration of infertility prior to surgery to be an inverse variable to success, and found the same relationship for increasing age. In 63 women who failed to conceive in a 2-4 year follow-up, 18 were married to men with adverse seminal parameters.

The report by Gordts et al[313] et al is of particular interest because it focused on 176 women having microsurgery for endometriosis. The entire gamut of mircrosurgical technique was employed with fine (8-0) suture, peritoneal grafts where necessary, etc. No difference in pregnancy rate at two years was noted by AFS staging. The authors concluded that this finding proved the value of a microsurgical approach to severe endometriosis, but other interpretations are possible, especially given the relatively low success rate in mild disease (43%).

If laparoscopy has any advantage over laparotomy in terms of eventual pregnancy rate, surely a major component must be avoidance of serosal drying and abrasion. Therefore, at laparotomy, probably the most important thing to do is to make an assiduous effort to employ constant irrigation and to avoid sponging of serosal surfaces. Our preferred irrigant is warmed lactated Ringer's solution with 5000 units of heparin per liter and epinephrine 1:600,000 to reduce clot formation and small vessel oozing, respectively. Cold solutions (i.e. room temperature) favor tissue ischemia from intense vasoconstriction. Alterations in tubal-ovarian anatomic juxtaposition and tubal distortion from adhesive bands is thought to be a factor in endometriosis-associated infertility in AFS stages III and IV in particular. Therefore, considerable effort should be made to restore normal anatomic relationships when surgery by any route is performed to enhance fertility.

Buttram[317] reported on a modified surgical technique for endometriosis therapy which stressed removal of diseased adnexae in the case of unilateral involvement. Illustrated specifics of uterosacral plication and round ligament suspension appear in that article.

Rock et al[318] examined the effect of ancillary procedures such as appendectomy, presacral neurectomy and/or uterine suspension on pregnancy rates after laparotomy and concluded that there was no statistical effect.

Pittaway[319] noted that occult endometrial implants were found in 38% of grossly normal appendices removed at laparotomy done for endometriosis but concluded that routine removal of that organ was not indicated for infertile patients.

Laparoscopy

Chong et al[320] reported a small series of patients with severe endometriosis managed by CO_2 laser laparoscopy (11) or by CO_2 laser laparotomy (13) in a non-randomized fashion at two centers. Pregnancy rates were 54.5% and 53.8%, respectively, along with the obvious decreased hospital stay and quicker recovery for the endoscopic group. A study by Fayez and Collazo[121] compared laparotomy to laparoscopy with all subjects receiving post operative danazol; the laparoscopy patients had superior pregnancy rates. Paulson et al[235] noted an 81% pregnancy rate in 181 patients having laser laparoscopy, 47% (9/19) for laparoscopy with electrosurgery, and 84% (97/116) pregnancy rate for patients managed by conservative laparotomy for AFS stages I and II. Controls managed expectantly had a 57% pregnancy rate (16/28). The difference between electrosurgery (ES) and laser (L) laparoscopy may be a function of gross disparity in sample size but certainly for the laser group laparoscopy was as efficacious as laparotomy and obviously less expensive. An excellent review by Cook and Rock[321] examined the role of laparoscopy in endometriosis diagnosis and therapy. Diagnosis of nonpigmented lesions which are more mitotically active than the more distinctive pigmented lesions, and careful search for deep seated ovarian endometriomas was stressed.

Adhesiolysis can be accomplished laparoscopically with blunt dissection, sharp dissection, ES or L. While one could selectively quote literature to support a particular bias, the truth is that neither the animal research data nor human experience has a consensus favoring any laser as clearly superior. Damage to adjacent organs can occur with mechanical sharp dissection as well as with energy methods. Endometriomas of the ovary rarely shell out intact. Entry and drainage of cyst contents with pelvic lavage allows for subsequent stripping of the capsule in most cases. Less tedious, and just as efficacious, in my opinion, is destruction of the capsule in situ with the YAG laser sapphire probe.

Deep lesions can be palpated indirectly at laparoscopy with simple probes and use of a YAG laser here is particularly appropriate because of its ability to deeply penetrate tissue. Pure vaporization is best accomplished with the CO_2 laser. Nezhat et al[119] compared CO_2, argon and KTP/532 lasers for laparoscopic therapy of endometriosis and concluded that the CO_2 laser was superior for relief of pain and for restoration of fertility. Keye et al[120] were the first to report a sizable argon laser series and like others, found that most pregnancies occurred within six months of surgery.

Reich and Mc Glynn[122] described their technique(s) of treatment for ovarian endometriosis using fulguration and excision. Daniell et al[322] described a technique of management using various lasers to incise and destroy the cyst wall coupled with a capsule stripping technique when possible. Twelve of 32 conceived following this surgery, and two more conceived after a second-look procedure. The multicentric study group[125] confirmed the efficacy of laparoscopy and documented health cost savings compared with laparotomy. Ultrasonography preoperatively is very helpful even if laparoscopy is scheduled. Small cystic teratomas deep in the ovary may be difficult to diagnose laparoscopically but have an almost pathognomonic ultrasound appearance. Septated cystic lesions alert the operator to the possibility of a diagnosis of ovarian neoplasia. Candiani et al[323] demonstrated the need for aggressive examination of the ovary by laparoscopic needle puncture to diagnose deep endometriomas in the absence of surface lesions. Preoperative transvaginal ultrasonography was helpful in detecting these lesions.

Comparison of literature results for laser laparoscopy and for electrosurgery suffers from the usual vagaries of this type of meta analysis - different classification systems, different populations, different surgical techniques and postoperative enhancing therapies, but these are the best data available. Some studies differentiate between patients having endometriosis without other adverse fertility factors. Gast et al[324] found that the presence of additional diagnoses such as cervical factor, seminal deficiency, and luteal phase disorders significantly decreased pregnancy rates following laser treatment of endometriosis. Murphy et al[325] noted a similar effect of other factors on fertility following ES therapy of endometriosis (seminal problems excluded). Treated anovulation had essentially no effect on pregnancy rate following surgery.

Electrosurgery (ES)

ES or fulguration was used laparoscopically for endometriosis as reported first by Eward in 1978[326]. Other reports followed, few with expectant management as controls, and some with danazol treatment as a comparison group. Table 21 shows some of these data segregated by severity although the classification systems are not uniform.

There is a feeling among surgeons that because laser energy can be better targeted to delivery at a discrete locus, and because there is no election flow to a dispersive electrode along tissue planes, laser is inherently safer than unipolar ES. This is probably true but is unsubstantiated by any actual experimental data. The Nowroozi[329] study is noteworthy because a true control group of laparoscopically verified, but not treated, endometriotic women was established. In eight months the treated group had a 61% pregnancy rate, but only 10 of 54 (19%) of controls had conceived. Sulewski et al[327] noted that 73% of conceptions following ES occurred within six months and 88% within 12. The Seiler study [328] found a 44% pregnancy rate at seven months with ES versus 39% for danazol treated patients with mild disease in a randomized protocol.

The Murphy study[325] is of interest because in addition to crude pregnancy rate data, life table analysis with a two-parameter experimental method was used as an ultra sophisticated statistical approach to follow-up.

Laser Laparoscopy

The CO_2 laser has a longer history of laparoscopic use than the newer flexible fiber lasers and therefore will be discussed in greater detail.

Kelly and Roberts[330] had an early report (1983) on use of CO_2 laser delivered via laparoscopy for treatment of endometriosis. Six of ten patients in their initial report conceived with three having a successful conception. Table 22 contains data from "pure" series, i.e. those in which perioperative drug therapy was not employed.

TABLE 21
PREGNANCY FOLLOWING LAPAROSCOPIC ELECTROSURGICAL DESTRUCTION OF ENDOMETRIOSIS

Author	No. Preg/No. Treated Stage				Follow-up Mos.
	Minimal	Mild %	Moderate	Severe	
Eward[326]	4/7 (57)	10/18 (56)			13
Sulewski et al[327]		20/42 (48)	20/58 (35)		37
Seiler et al[328]		20/45 (44)			7
Nowroozi et al[329]		42/69 (61)			
Murphy et al[325]	24/36 (67)	18/36 (50)	2/7 (29)	0/30 (0)	8
Total	28/43 (65)	120/210 (57)	22/65 (34)	0/30 (0)	

- Comparison of Tables 21 and 22 shows that there is no real difference in pregnancy rates between ES and L for stages I and II of endometriosis. But there seems to be an advantage favoring L in more advanced stages as suggested by this meta analysis.

- Noteworthy also is the trend toward diminution of pregnancy rate differences according to stage in patients having CO_2 laser laparoscopy
- Most authors reported a trend towards most pregnancies occurring within the first six to eight months following surgery.

Olive and Martin[338] used different sophisticated statistical models to demonstrate an immediate, albeit transient, effect of laser

TABLE 22
PREGNANCY RATES AFTER LAPAROSCOPIC CO_2 LASER TREATMENT OF ENDOMETRIOSIS

	No. Pregnant/No. Treated Stage				Follow-up Mos.
Author	Minimal	Mild	Moderate	Severe	
Kelly and Roberts[330]	3/3 (100)	3/7 (43)			6
Feste[331]	24/47 (51)	4/6 (66)	2/5 (40)		12
Martin[332]	25/56 (45)	22/45 (49)	9/14 (64)		12
Davis[333]	----	20/31 (65)*	15/26 (58)	2/7 (29)	15
Donnez[334]**	26/42 (62)	11/21 (52)	3/7 (43)		18
Sutton and Hill[335] #	15/16 (94)	17/25 (68)	11/13 (85)	2/2 (100)	6-72
Gast et al[324]	36/70 (51)	12/33 (38)	9/19 (47)		10
Fayez et al[336]	27/38 (71)	33/44 (75)			12
Nezhat et al[337]#	28/39 (72)	60/86 (70)	45/67 (6)	35/51 (69)	
Paulson et al[235]	109/140 (78)	60/88 (68)			8-32
TOTAL	293/451 (65)	242/386 (62)	95/151 (62)	39/60 (65)	

* Minimal and mild combined

Patients with additional fertility factors eliminated from study.

** Ovarian endometrioma limited to 3 cm.

laparoscopy on fecundity in endometriosis patients. Subgroups of patients with additional diagnoses, and those treated pharmacologically were evaluated. Stage had no effect on predicted pregnancy rate up to three years following surgery. Monthly fecundity was unaffected by subgroups. Fecundity was similar for those treated by laser laparoscopy, danazol, expectant management and laparotomy for stages I and II.

Argon Laser

Following experimental work in the rabbit[339], Keye et al[120] published a series on use of the argon laser in humans with endometriosis. This particular laser has the advantage of color-seeking selective absorption (provided the lesions are pigmented) but has not gained in popularity over the other lasers for treatment of endometriosis. This is probably because the argon laser has a relatively low maximum output which makes eradication of deep lesions difficult. Nevertheless, Badawy et al[340] reported a 42% pregnancy rate in 31 patients treated with this modality.

YAG Laser

Lomano[341] used the neodynium:yttrium aluminum-garnet (Nd:YAG) laser as a bare fiber

TABLE 23
COMPARISON OF CO_2 AND YAG LASERS

	CO_2	YAG (Sapphire Probe)
Delivery System	Rigid Arm	Flexible Fiber
Absorption by Water	Great	Minimal
Mirror Alignment	Frequent	Rare
Smoke Production	Great	Minimal
Delivery Mode	Focussed Beam Non-touch	Touch
Vaporization	Excellent	Marginal
Coagulation	Minimal	Excellent
Lateral Tissue Damage	Minimal	Moderate
Distal Tissue Damage	Moderate	Minimal

laparoscopically for endometriosis in conjunction with postoperative danazol. Since that report all other authors have stressed use of the distal sapphire probe or sculptured tips to focus energy at the tip which avoids the shotgun scatter pattern of the bare fiber which might lead to inadvertant damage of adjacent organs.

The KTP/532 laser has half the wave length of the YAG laser, and in general, has similar tissue effects. Table 23 compares the YAG laser and CO_2 laser systems. The sapphire probe or specific sculptured tip chosen determines the geometry of the lesion. Our group has reported a continuous series of patients treated with the YAG laser sapphire probe laparoscopically[342-344]. For 126 consecutive endometriosis patients desiring fertility, rates were 14/19 (74%), 21/36 (58%), 29/36 (42%) and 9/35 (26%) by stages I-IV respectively. Most of these patients were referrals who had failed to conceive with previous pharmacologic or surgical therapy. Duration of infertility was 51 months. Figure 29 (A-D) demonstrates our technique of in situ destruction of endometriotic ovarian cysts. Copious lavage with an adequate aspirator-irrigator using warmed physiologic solution is necessary. We favor (obviously) an instrument of our own design.* Other authors[345-346] have found the YAG laser efficacious in treating endometriosis.

(* Corson Aspirator/Irrigator, Cabot-Medical)

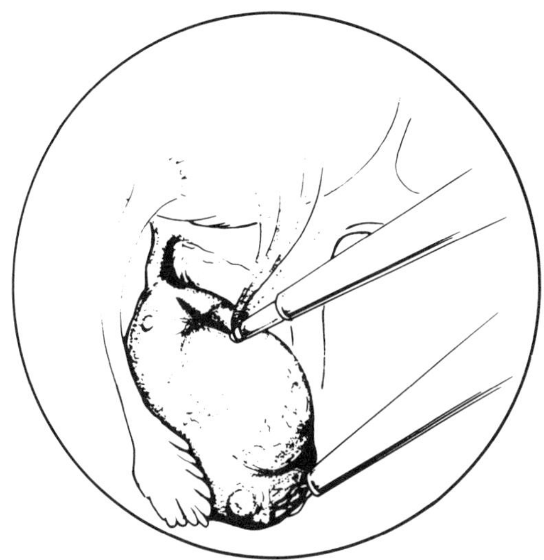

Fig. 29A The ovary is grasped and the cyst entered using the sapphire probe.

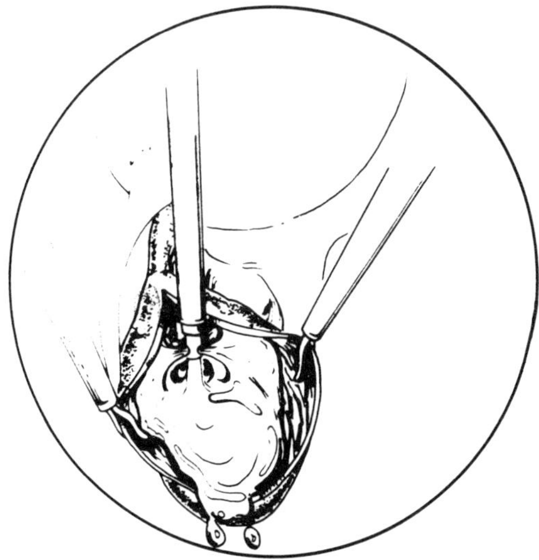

Fig. 29B The irrigator aspirator is used to wash out the cyst and to enable the cyst wall to be examined.

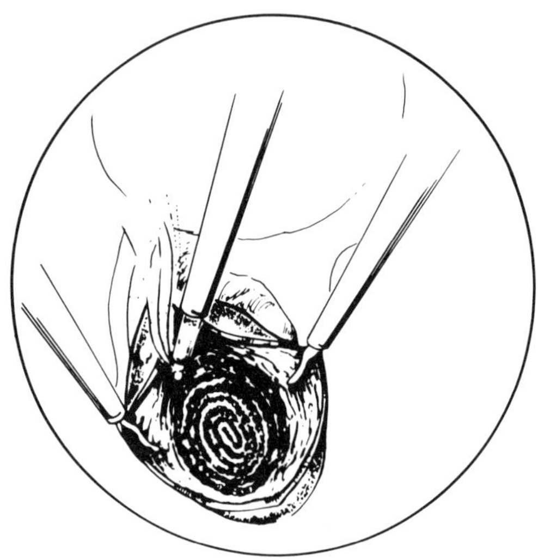

Fig. 29C The chisel tip sapphire probe is used to destroy the cyst wall in situ starting from the bottom and moving toward the top in a spiral like fashion.

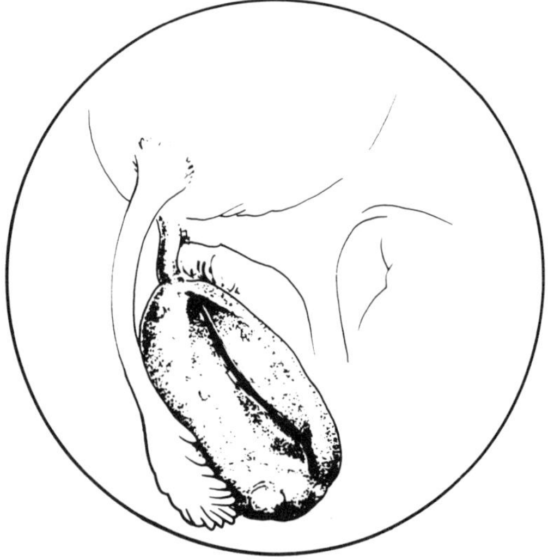

Fig. 29D The edges fold toward each other and no suturing is necessary.

Notes

#22 SUPEROVULATION

Dodson et al[347] reported a landmark series in which superovulation with hMG/hCG was used empirically with intrauterine insemination (IUI) for a group of infertile patients including 55 with endometriosis in the absence of ovulatory, uterine or seminal pathology. The duration of infertility for all the patients studied was 5.3 years, but a specific duration for the endometriotic sub-group was not given. The patients with endometriosis had minimal findings in 13, mild disease in 27, moderate pathology in 13, and two were in the severe group. A program of four treatment cycles was offered, but no pregnancy ensued after the second cycle. Fecundity was 0.17 for these patients, divided as 0.40 for minimal endometriosis, 0.12 for mild disease, 0.17 for moderate and 0 for the severe cases. The multiple pregnancy rate for endometriotic patients was not specified.

Corson et al[348] reported on a series of 302 patients in 991 cycles of IUI with and without concomitant superovulation, with 89 having endometriosis (43, 26, 20, 5 in stages I-IV, respectively). Analysis showed no difference in post coital test results or in the presence of cervical factors for this group versus the other diagnostic categories. Monthly fecundity was 0.12 for minimal endometriosis with hMG/IUI, 0.06 for mild disease and 0.03 for moderate-severe findings, compared with 0.10 for the entire study group and compared also with 0.01 for untreated cycles. IUI alone had no statistical effect compared with no treatment at all.

Deaton et al[349] used a randomized prospective protocol of clomiphene citrate stimulation coupled with IUI in a group of endometriotic patients (27) who had not conceived following surgical therapy. Patients were randomized to four cycles of treatment or observation with a crossover to the other arm of the study if pregnancy did not occur. Seven pregnancies occurred in 72 treated cycles (fecundity of 0.09) versus five of 150 control cycles (0.03). Possible mechanisms explaining the seemingly beneficial response to superovulation either with or without IUI include changes in ovulatory parameters, direct and indirect hormonal events and effect on sperm transport.

- First, there is an increase of oocytes available for tubal capture, fertilization, and nidation, with all of these steps possibly being compromised by even minimal endometriosis. Whether the quality of these oocytes is improved by programs of superovulation remains to be seen.

- Second, estrogen levels are undoubtedly higher than in natural cycles and some benefit may accrue from this. For instance, these high levels favor increase in quantity and quality of mucus, not only that which is sampled at the external cervical os, but along the entire internal reproductive tract. Thus, sperm transport may be improved.

- Many clinicians routinely and prophylactically utilize progesterone for luteal support in stimulated cycles, so that this may be an indirect hormonal effect.

While we[348] could not demonstrate a beneficial effect of IUI in the absence of cervical or seminal pathology, over and above that seen with hMG alone, IUI certainly delivers a number of actively motile sperm into the uterine cavity far greater than that achieved with coitus.

The number of treatment cycles over which this non-specific and certainly empiric therapy should be given before moving on to even more aggressive treatment depends on the usually encountered factors of female age, duration of infertility, and the anxiety level of the couple. In addition, one must consider the added factor of cost, since few medical insurance programs cover all of the ancillary charges including laboratory fees, costs of multiple ultrasonic examinations and especially the cost of gonadotropins.

Our own philosophy is one of recommending three to six cycles of super-ovulation with or without IUI depending on all of the above factors. We also skip cycles between treatments with hMG. This schema allows for regression of ovarian enlargement and luteal cysts seen commonly with this therapy, and also seems to lessen the stress on the couple.

Notes

#23 ASSISTED REPRODUCTION

In 1983, Mahadevan et al[350] reported on an in vitro fertilization (IVF) experience with patients in various diagnostic groups. No difference in pregnancy rate for endometriotic patients was noted compared with other groups. Another Australian IVF practice reported a pregnancy rate of 18% for women with tubal disease versus 13%, 14%, 6% and 2% for stages I-IV of endometriosis, respectively[351], with totals of 15, 25, 26 and 30 patients by stage over 154 treatment cycles. Oocyte recovery and fertilization rates were unaffected by endometriosis except for a reduced number of developed follicles and retrieved follicles in stages III and IV.

By far, the most intensive study of IVF for treatment of resistant endometriosis-associated infertility has been made by the Norfolk group[352-354]. In the last report Oehninger and Rosenwaks extended the study to cover 165 patients between 1981 through 1988 in 341 cycles of IVF. Of special interest was their Group I patients (25 in 59 cycles) with a history of endometriosis diagnosed previously by laparoscopy but who had no evidence of endometriosis at laparoscopic egg retrieval. Group II patients-108 in 227 cycles-had stage I or II endometriosis and Group III-32 patients in 55 cycles-had stage III or IV disease diagnosed at the time of retrieval. Stimulation protocols changed slightly over the years of the study but this was not a selective factor by group. As with the Australian data, more oocytes were recovered for Groups I and II and a greater number of preovulatory oocytes were obtained than for the patients with advanced disease. Fertilization of preovulatory oocytes was not different by group. While transfer rates were similar, group III had fewer total embryos replaced. Progesterone levels in the luteal phase were similar by group.

No differences in pregnancy rates or ongoing pregnancy were apparent by group (Table 24). Therefore, neither the fertilization rate, cleavage rate, pregnancy rate nor ongoing pregnancy rate was adversely affected by endometriosis.

Hulme et al[355] reported a series of 46 patients with endometriosis treated with gamete intrafallopian transfer (GIFT) within a total group of 464 GIFT cycles, with an overall pregnancy rate of 24%. Mean age for endometriotic patients was 31 years and mean duration of infertility was 5 years. Mean AFS score was 13 (range 1-40).

TABLE 24*
IVF PREGNANCY RATES FOR ENDOMETRIOTIC PATIENTS BY TRANSFER

	GROUP I (HISTORY ONLY)	GROUP II (STAGE I/II)	GROUP III (STAGE III/IV)
		(%)	
PREGNANT	16	26	28
ON-GOING	13	15	12

* Adapted form Oehninger and Rosenwaks[354].

- The pregnancy rate for the endometriotic patients in this study was 31% per cycle (18/59).

- 15 pregnancies resulted in 22 live born deliveries with one set of quadruplets resulting from the placement of four oocytes in all cases.

- There was one spontaneous abortion, one interruption of pregnancy with Downs syndrome and one ectopic pregnancy.

- In 24 of 46 cycles a seminal factor was also diagnosed. Ongoing pregnancy rate here was 28% versus 26% (including the Downs syndrome) for the normospermic endometriosis patients.

- In 11 patients ovarian endometriomas were aspirated during the GIFT procedure with four of those patients conceiving. No active therapy was performed other than aspiration.

Gindoff et al[356] reported a mixed series of IVF and GIFT patients in whom lysis of adhesions or "fulguration" of endometriosis was performed concomitantly in 19 versus 13 who had no active operative intervention other than egg retrieval by laparoscopy. The clinical pregnancy rate was 25% for the actively treated group and 30% for the other.

Remorgida et al[357] reported on using GnRH-a for six months prior to GIFT stimulation in stages I and II endometriosis, versus using a flare-up (short GnRH-a protocol) and results were compared with a standard stimulation protocol. Pregnancy rates were 56%, 32% and 33%, respectively (n=18, 19, 18 by group).

Batzofin et al[358] used concomitant CO_2 or Argon laser therapy at GIFT (27) and IVF (2) in 29 women with 26 having active endometriosis with a mean duration of infertility of 3.4 years.

- In the 26 with endometriosis 15 intrauterine (58%) and 3 ectopic pregnancies were reported.
- Ten of the 15 pregnancies were ongoing to the point of viability.
- The ongoing pregnancy rate was similar to a control group not using laser therapy.
- Three of four patients with severe endometriosis conceived with all three delivering.
- The ongoing pregnancy rate in this study was similar to a control group (34% successful pregnancies) who were not treated actively during oocyte retrieval.

Corson et al[236] reported a series of 77 women in 92 cycles of GIFT in which CO_2 or YAG laser therapy was employed during the procedure in 20 cycles, electrosurgery in 28 cycles and no active intervention in 44. Table 25 shows pertinent data:

- Pregnancy rates in stage III especially were impressive whether active therapy or only egg retrieval and gamete transfer alone was employed.

- AFS score had no effect on total oocyte recovery.

- In patients having more than one procedure (nine with two procedures and three with three attempts) AFS scores were restaged. Staging was unchanged in four patients having no active therapy. Of six patients with electrosurgery, four were unchanged at the second procedure and two were reduced within a few months from the initial operation. One laser patient who had a second procedure had a reduction from stage II to zero.

These results document the beneficial effect of assisted reproduction for resistant infertility associated with endometriosis. In addition, our findings demonstrate the rapidity with which endometriosis can recur following apparently successful therapy, since repeat GIFT procedures usually were performed within a few months of the first.

Dispiriting was our observation that in 44 patients followed for a mean of 14 months following GIFT with 24 having active operative intervention, only two pregnancies occurred; one with superovulation and IUI and one with IVF. This finding was at odds with data reported by Damewood and Rock[359] who found a 28% pregnancy rate at 10 months in 39 patients who had active intervention during a laparoscopic retrieval for endometriosis which did not result in pregnancy during that cycle.

In summary, both IVF and GIFT would appear to offer benefit for patients with endometriosis who have not conceived with less invasive methods of therapy after long-term infertility. While it is not yet clear whether active operative intervention during oocyte collection has a salutary effect on pregnancy rate, it certainly does not exert a deleterious one. Bulky, stimulated ovaries may present some considerable difficulty to treatment of endometriosis, and only skilled laparoscopists should consider concomitant treatment of endometriosis at the time of oocyte retrieval.

TABLE 25
PREGNANCY RATES IN GIFT CYCLES ACCORDING TO ADDITIONAL SURGICAL TREATMENT DURING OOCYTE RETRIEVAL

	American Fertility Society Score									
	All Cycles		I		II		II		IV	
Total	n	(% Pregnant)	n	(% Pregnant)	n	(% Pregnant)	n	(% Pregnant)	n	(% Pregnant)
All	92	(35)	36	(47)	35	(14)	19	(53)	2	(0)
Fulguration	28	(25)	1	(100)	19	(16)	7	(43)	1	(0)
Laser	20	(45)	3	(67)	8	(25)	9	(56)	0	(0)
No Treatment	44	(36)	32	(44)	8	(0)	3	(67)	1	(0)

From Corson SL, Batzer FR, Gocial B, Daly DC, Eisenberg E, Huppert LC, Maislin G: Surgical treatment of endometriosis at the time of gamete intrafallopian transfer. J. Reprod Med 36:274, 1991. Reproduced with permission from the Journal of Reproductive Medicine.

Notes

#24 RECURRENT ENDOMETRIOSIS

A clinical dictum states that women who conceive following therapy for endometriosis are less likely to have clinically obvious recurrence of the disease process. Of course this is an ad hoc, propter hoc argument. True, the hormonal changes which occur naturally during pregnancy form the basis upon which pseudopregnancy was advanced as therapy. Also true is the fact that at cesarean section, previously active lesions seem to be atrophic or "burned-out". But cases are on record of endometriosis actually worsening during pregnancy. Most important, patients who conceive after any therapy may simply be those with a greater reduction of active lesions having nothing to do with subsequent pregnancy-mediated hormonal events. Doctors and patients alike know that endometriosis has a reputation for recrudescence, but to what extent?

Schenken and Malinak[316] addressed this issue by following 117 patients for three years after a conservative laparotomy.

- Another operation was necessary in 28 (21%) during this interval for return of pain or continued infertility.
- But the rate of reoperation was 41% for those not conceiving after the initial surgery versus only 4% who had become pregnant during that interval.
- Conception then occurred in 12% (3/26) following the second procedure.

- An equal number (3) had total abdominal hysterectomy as a third operation.

- Initial staging showed that the more advanced cases were more likely to have a second procedure, but the interval to this second surgery was not related to the degree of staging.

The study of Rock et al[311] done at Johns Hopkins noted a 13.5% reoperation rate during a variable interval of follow-up. But 30% had return of symptoms thought to be due to endometriosis.

As mentioned in the previous section[236], we noted recurrence of active endometriosis only months after laser surgery in patients having a GIFT procedure. The trend towards conservative adnexal therapy by any route may predispose to recrudescence, especially if the ovary is "peppered" with implants. Sound surgical judgement is needed to decide whether removal of such an ovary at the time of the primary procedure is preferable to an attempt at ovarian conservation.

24.

Punnonen et al[360] noted a reoperation rate of 15% (132/903) in surgically treated endometriosis in a 6-10 year follow-up, with seven patients having the second procedure within one year, 91 at 1-5 years, and 34 after the fifth year.

Candiani et al[361] examined the results of repetitive conservative surgery in 42 patients with endometriosis. Stages were, Stages I - II (3 patients), Stage III (25), and 14 women were Stage IV. The mean follow-up was 42 months.

- Pain of one pattern or another returned in 19%, all of whom had pain as a presenting symptom prior to the repeat procedure (none had been treated with pre-sacral neurectomy).

- Pregnancy occurred in 8/28 (29%) with a cumulative pregnancy rate of 31% at 27 months.

- A third operation was necessary in six patients, with a mean interval of 35 months.

Wheeler and Malinak[367] surveyed the literature in 1983 and noted a recurrence rate of 17% to 29% after pseudopregnancy alone as therapy; and a 39% recurrence after danazol treatment. Surgical therapy was followed by recurrence in 2% through 47%. Andrews and Larsen[85] reported a 36% recurrence after combined pseudopregnancy-surgery therapy. Wheeler and Malinak used 45 non-reoperated women followed for five years as controls against the reoperated endometriotic patients who were further divided according to whether endometriosis was actually found at the time of the second procedure.

- From an initial sample of 423 women, 62 (15%) had another procedure.

- Annual recurrence ranged from 0.9% in the first year to 14% in the eighth year.

- Cumulative 3- and 5- year recurrence rates were 14% and 40%, respectively.

- Mean time to reoperation was 35 months.

- Staging was not indicative of recurrence risks.

- Pregnancy was achieved by 47% after the second procedure.

- Pregnancy after the first operation delayed but did not prevent against recurrence.

- In the reoperated group of patients, 20% required a third procedure.

- Of the 62 reoperated patients, 21 had no identifiable endometriosis at the time of the second procedure. Diagnoses in these patients were: adhesions (10), adhesions and tubal pregnancies (7), leiomyoma (2) and normal pelvis (2).

Summary

- The recurrence rate for endometriosis severe enough to warrant reoperation after initial conservative laparotomy is approximately 15% in the first three to five years depending upon whether the indication for repeat surgery is return of pain or continued infertility.

- With respect to continued infertility, IVF and/or GIFT may be more commonly substituted as a secondary procedure.

- Results of operative laparoscopy and recurrence have not been adequately evaluated.

- The outlook for pregnancy following a second procedure is not so bleak as previously assumed.

- Recurrence rates after medical therapy are higher and symptoms of pain reoccur more promptly than with conservative laparotomy (see also discussion on pain control).

- There is no evidence that combined medical-surgical approaches, in either order, affect recurrence rates.

- The consensus is that ovarian endometriosis, in particular, is best treated surgically.

- When symptoms return following surgery, medical treatment may be helpful as a delaying tactic, especially if the patient is willing to have repeated courses of such treatment employed on an interval basis as needed.

- Preoperative treatment with hormonally active agents may also be of help in reducing the size of lesions and in reduction of inflammatory adhesions.

Notes

#25 SUMMARY

I know of no clinical entity in all of gynecology whose diagnosis and treatment is predicated on less firm scientific data than endometriosis. Indeed, its pathophysiology, morphology and mechanisms of pain production as well as causation of infertility seem to become more varied and complex as new information accumulates. At the same time that patients clamor for laser laparoscopy or treatment with the newest GnRH-a agent, statistical studies support a certain degree of therapeutic nihilism for minimal and/or mild disease. The currently employed staging system often has little correlation with endometriosis-induced pain, since the pain is frequently more related to the location of the lesions rather than to the extent or volume of the implants. Many studies, in addition, have generated results in which the pregnancy rate was not really proportionate to the staging.

Through the fog, there are patches where data seem to allow for some conclusions of some validity.

- Operative laparoscopy is as efficacious as laparotomy for restoration of fertility.

- Lasers are helpful but probably add little to fertility rates compared with other methods of surgical destruction or extirpation of lesions.

- The GnRH-a drugs are at least as efficacious as danazol both for pain control and for fertility augmentation and offer a good alternative to patients who cannot tolerate danazol side-effects.

- Second operations are associated with a reasonable salvage of fertility.

- Superovulation with or without IUI is an empiric form of therapy which seems to have value, perhaps on a number of different fronts. It should probably be tried prior to advancement to assisted methods of reproduction provided there is no strong tubal component.

- Assisted reproductive techniques such as IVF and GIFT further boost pregnancy yield in cases resistant to drug or surgical treatment.

There is no single, direct therapeutic approach to endometriosis. Now that we have so many treatment options none of which is clearly superior to the others, physicians must spend considerable time in educating patients so that they can take part in the treatment formulation process.

Short of pharmacologic or surgical induction of permanent menopause, no treatment "cures" endometriosis reliably for the vast majority of patients, since the primary mechanisms of its formation remain uninterrupted, with the potential for exacerbation at any time. A magic therapeutic bullet is not on the immediate horizon. On an optimistic note, perusal of daily operative schedules leads one to conclude that fewer hysterectomies are performed for endometriosis than in years hence. Therefore, judicious choice of therapies and the willingness to employ repeat courses of pharmacologic agents or repeated laparoscopies offer considerable benefit to the patient both for pain control and fertility restoration.

Notes

BIBLIOGRAPHY

1. Janne O, Kauppila A, Kokko E, Lantto T, Ronnberg L, Vihko R: Estrogen and progestin receptors in endometriosis lesions: Comparison with endometrial tissue. Am J Obstet Gynecol 141:562, 1981.
2. Vihko R, Isotalo H, Kauppila a, et al: Hormonal regulation of endometrium and endometriosis. Raynaud JP (ed), Medical Management of Endometriosis, Raven Press, New York, pps. 79-89, 1984.
3. Dizerega GS, Barber DL, Hodgen GD: Endometriosis: Role of ovarian steroids in initiation, maintenance, and suppression. Fertil Steril 33:649, 1980.
4. Vasquez G, Cornillie F, Brosens IA: Peritoneal endometriosis: scanning electron microscopy and histology of minimal pelvic endometriotic lesions. Fertil Steril 42:696, 1984.
5. Jansen RPS, Russell P: Nonpigmented endometriosis: Clinical, laparoscopic, and pathologic definition. Am J Obstet Gynecol 155:1154, 1986.
6. Chatman DL, Zbella EA: Pelvic peritoneal defects and endometriosis: further observations. Fertil Steril 46:711, 1986.
7. Stripling MC, Martin DC, Poston WM: Does endometriosis have a typical appearance? J Reprod Med 33:879, 1988.
8. Stripling MC, Martin DC, Chatman DL, Zwaag RV, Poston WM: Subtle appearance of pelvic endometriosis. Fertil Steril 49:427, 1988.
9. Martin DC, Hubert GD, Levy BS: Depth of infiltration of endometriosis. J Gynecol Surg 5:55, 1989.
10. Nisolle M, Paindaveine B, Bourdon A, Berliere M, Casanas-Roux F, Donnez J: Histologic study of peritoneal endometriosis in infertile women. Fertil Steril 53:984, 1990.
11. Sampson JA: Peritoneal endometriosis due to the menstrual dissemination of endometrial tissue into the peritoneal cavity. Am J Obstet Gynecol 14:422, 1927.
12. Novak E: The significance of uterine mucosa in the fallopian tubes with a discussion of the origin of aberrant endometrium. Am J Obstet Gynecol 12:484, 1926.
13. Halban J: Hysteroadenosis Metastica. Wien Klin Wochenschr 37:12-5, 1924.

14. Fakih HN, Tamura R, Kesselman Am, DeCherney AH: Endometriosis after tubal ligation. J Reprod Med 30:939, 1985
15. Dodge ST, Pumphrey RS, Miyazawa K: Peritoneal endometriosis in women requesting reversal of serilization. Fertil Steril 45:774, 1986.
16. Sampson JA: Metastasis of embolic endometriosis due to menstrual dissemination of endometrial tissue into the venous circulation. Am J Pathol 3:93, 1927.
17. Halme J, Hammond MG, Hulka JF, Raj SG, Talbert LM: Retrograde menstruation in healthy women and in patients with endometriosis. Obstet Gynecol 64:151, 1984.
18. Ridley JH: The histogenesis of endometriosis: A review of facts and fancies. Obstet Gynecol Surv 23:1, 1968.
19. Cramer DW: Epidemiology of endometriosis. Tilson EA (ed), Endometriosis, Alan R. Liss, New York, pps. 5-22, 1987.
20. Cramer DW, Wilson E, Stillman RJ, Berger MJ, Belisle S, Schiff I, Albrecht B, Gibson M, Stadel BV, Schoenbaum SC: The relation of endometriosis to menstrual characteristics, smoking and exercise. JAMA 255:1904-1908.
21. Sanfilippo JS, Wakim NG, Schikler KN, Yussman MA: Endometriosis in association with uterine anomaly. Am J Obstet Gynecol 154:39, 1986.
22. Olive DL, Henderson DY: Endometriosis and Müllerian anomalies. Obstet Gynecol 69:412, 1987.
23. Stillman RJ, Miller LC: Diethylstilbestrol exposure in utero and endometriosis in infertile females. Fertil Steril 41:369, 1984.
24. Moen MH: Endometriosis in women at interval sterilization. Acta Obstet Gynecol Scand 66:451, 1987.
25. Strathy JH, Molgaard CA, Coulan CV and Metton LJ: Endometriosis and infertility: A laparoscopic survey of endometriosis among fertile and infertile women. Fertil Steril 38:667, 1982.
26. Duignan NM, Jordan JA, Coughlan BM, Logan-Edwards R: One thousand consecutive cases of diagnostic laparoscopy. J Obstet Gynaecol Br Commonw 79:1016, 1972.
27. Hasson HM: Incidence of endometriosis in diagnostic laparoscopy. J Reprod Med 16:135, 1976.
28. Kleppinger RK: One thousand laparoscopies at a community hospital. J Reprod Med 13:13, 1974.

29. Liston WA, Bradford WP, Downie J, Kerr MG: Laparoscopy in a general gynecologic unit. Am J Obstet Gynecol 113:672, 1972.
30. Peterson EP, Behrman SJ: Laparoscopy of the infertile patient. Obstet Gynecol 36:363, 1970.
31. Talbot HM, Leeton J: The role of laparoscopy in 1,400 patients. Med J Aust 1:36, 1974.
32. Houston DE, Noller KL, Melton LJ, Selwyn BJ, Hardy RJ: Incidence of pelvic endometriosis in Rochester, Minnesota, 1970-1079. Am J Epi 125:959, 1987.
33. Chatman DL, Ward AB: Endometriosis in adolescents. J Reprod Med 27:156, 1982.
34. Goldstein DP, deCholnoky C, Emans SJ, Leventhal JM: Laparoscopy in the diagnosis and management of pelvic pain in adolescents. J Reprod Med 24:251, 1980.
35. Simpson JL, Elias S, Malinak LR, Buttman VC: Heritable aspects of endometriosis. I. Genetic studies. Am J Obstet Gynecol 137:327, 1980.
36. Malinak LR, Buttram VC, Elias S, Simpson, JL: Heritable aspects of endometriosis. II. Clinical characteristics of familial endometriosis. Am J Obstet Gynecol 137:332, 1980.
37. Patton PE, Field CS, Harms RW, Coulam CB: CA-125 levels in endometriosis. Fertil Steril 45:770, 1986.
38. Pittaway DE, Fayez JA, Douglas JW: Serum CA-125 in the evaluation of benign adnexal cysts. Am J Obstet Gynecol 157:1426, 1987.
39. Dawood MY, Khan-Dawood FS, Ramos J: Plasma and peritoneal fluid levels of CA 125 in women with endometriosis. Am J Obstet Gynecol 159:1526, 1988.
40. Kauppila A, Telimaa, Ronnberg L, Vuori J: Placebo-controlled study on serum concentrations of CA-125 before and after treatment of endometriosis with danazol or high-dose medroxyprogesterone acetate alone or after surgery. Fertil Steril 49:37, 1988.
41. Fedele L, Arcaina L, Vercellini P, Bianchi S, Candiani GB: Serum CA 125 measurements in the diagnosis of endometriosis recurrence. Obstet Gynecol 72:19, 1988.
42. Moloney MD, Thornton JG, Cooper EH: Serum CA 125 antigen levels and disease severity in patients with endometriosis. Obstet Gynecool 73:767, 1989.
43. Pittaway DE: The use of serial CA 125 concentrations to monitor endometriosis in infertile women. Am J Obstet Gynecol 163:1032, 1990.
44. Lehtovirta P, Apter D, Stenman UH: Serum CA 125 levels during menstrual cycles. Br J Obstet Gynaecol 97:930, 1990.

45. Sampson JA: Endometrial carcinoma of the ovary arising in endometrial tissue in that organ. Arch Surg 10:1, 1925.
46. Moll UM, Chumas JC, Chalas E, Mann WJ: Ovarian carcinoma arising in atypical endometriosis. Obstet Gynecol 75:537, 1990.
47. Heapes JM, Nieberg RK, Berek JS: Malignant neoplasms arising in endometriosis. Obstet Gynecol 75:1023, 1990
48. Reimnitz C, Brand E, Nieberg RK, Hacker NF: Malignancy arising in endometriosis associated with unopposed estrogen replacement. Obstet Gynecol 71:444, 1988.
49. Revised American Fertility Society Classification of Endometriosis. Fertil Steril 43:351, 1985.
50. Classification of endometriosis. American Fertility Society. Fertil Steril 32:633, 1979.
51. Acosta AA, Buttram VC, Franklin RR, Besch PK: Proposed classification of pelvic endometriosis. Obstet Gynecol 42:19, 1973.
52. Jenkins S, Olive DL, Haney AF: Endometriosis: Pathogenic Implications of the Anatomic Distribution. Obstet Gynecol 67:335, 1986.
53. Fedele L, Parazzini F, Bianchi S, Arcaini L, Candiani GB: Stage and localization of pelvic endometriosis and pain. Fertil Steril 53:155, 1990.
54. Luciano AA, Pitkin RM: Endometriosis: approaches to diagnosis and treatment. Surgery Annual: 1984, Nyhus L (ed), Appleton Crofts, Norwalk, CT, pps 297-312, 1984.
55. Rovati V, Faleschini E, Vercellini P, Nervetti G, Tagliabue G, Benzi G: Endometrioma of the liver. Am J Obstet Gynecol 163:1490, 1990.
56. Mac Afee CHG, Greer HL: Intestinal endometriosis. J Obstet Gynecol Br Emp 67:539, 1960.
57. Stahl C, Grimes EM: Endometriosis of the small bowel. Case reports and review of the literature. Obstet Gynecol Surgey 42:131, 1987.
58. Meyers WC, Kelvin FM, Jones RS: Diagnosis and surgical treatment of colonic endometriosis. Arch Surg 114:169, 1979.
59. Floberg J. Backdahl M. Silfersward C, Thomassen PA: Postpartum performation of the colon due to endometriosis. Acta Obstet Cynecol Scand 63:183, 1984.
60. Weed JC, Ray JE: Endometriosis of the bowel. Obstet Gynecol 69:727, 1987.

61. Badawy SZA, Freedman L, Numann P, Bonaventura M, Kim S: Diagnosis and management of intestinal endometriosis. A report of five cases. J Reprod Med 33:851, 1988.
62. Coronado C, Franklin RR, Lotze EC, Bailey HR, Valdes CT: Surgical treatment of symtomatic colorectal endometriosis. Fertil Steril 53:411, 1990.
63. Laube DW, Calderwood GW, Benda JA: Endometriosis causing ureteral obstruction. Obstet Gynecol 65:69S, 1985.
64. Maxson WS, Hill GA, Herbert CM, Kaufman AJ, Pittaway DE, Daniell JF, Winfield AC, Wentz AC: Ureteral abnormalities in women with endometriosis. Fertil Steril 46:1159, 1986.
65. Claman P, Taymor ML, Berger MJ, Seibel MM: Danazol therapy for proximal obstruction of the oviduct. J Reprod Med 31:687, 1986.
66. Rivlin ME, Krueger RP, Wiser WL: Danazol in the management of ureteral obstruction secondary to endometriosis. Fertil Steril 44:274, 1985.
67. Matsuura K, Kawasaki N, Oka M, Ii H, Maeyama M: Treatment with danazol of ureteral obstruction caused by endometriosis. Acta Obstet Scand 64:339, 1985.
68. Bergquist A, Bergquist D, Lindholm K, Linell F: Endometriosis in the uterosacral ligament giving orthopedic symptoms through compression of the sciatic nerve and surgically treated via an extraperitoneal approach keeping the pelvic organs intact. Acta Obstet Gynecol Scand 66:93, 1987.
69. Redwine DB, Sharpe DR: Endometriosis of the obturator nerve. A case report. J Reprod Med 35:434, 1990.
70. Foster DC, Stern JL, Buscema J, REock JA, Woodruff JD: Pleural and parenchymal plumonary endometriosis. Obstet Gynecol 58:552, 1981.
71. Johnson WM, Tyndal CM: Pulmonary endometriosis: treatment with danazol. Obstet Gynecol 69:506, 1987.
72. Suginami H, Hamada K, Yano K: A case of endometriosis of the lung treated with danazol. 66:68S, 1985.
73. Steck WD, Helwig EB: Cutaneous Endometriosis. JAMA 191:101, 1965.
74. Lundstrom V, Green K. Svanborg K: Endogenous prostaglandins, indomethacin and dysmenorrhea. Prostaglandinc 11:893, 1976.
75. Yikorkala O, Viinikka L: Prostaglandins and endometriosis. Acta Obstet Gynecol Scand (suppl) 113:105, 1983.

76. Corson SL, Bolognese RJ: Ibuprofen therapy for dysmenorrhea. J Reprod Med 20:246, 1978.
77. Chan WY, Dawood MY, Fuchs F: Relief of dysmenorrhea with the prostaglandin synthetase inhibitor ibuprofen: Effect on prostaglandin levels in mentrual fluid. 135:102, 1979.
78. Henzl MR, Izu A: Naproxen and naproxen sodium in dysmenorrhea: Development from in vitro inhibition of prostaglandin synthesis to suppression of uterine contractions in women and demonstration of clinical efficacy. Acta Obstet Gynecol Scand Suppl 87:105, 1979.
79. Chan WY, Fuchs F, Powell AM: Effects of naproxen sodium on mentrual prostaglandins and primary dysmenorrhea. Obstet Gynecol 61:285, 1983.
80. Kauppila A, Ronnberg L: Naproxen sodium in dysmenorrhea secondary to endometriosis. Obstet Gynecol 65:379, 1985.
81. Nisolle-Pochet M, Casanas-Roux F, Donnez J: Histologic study of ovarian endometriosis after hormonal therapy. Fertil Steril 49:423:1988.
82. Kistner RW: The treatment of endometriosis inducing pseudopregnancy with ovarian hormones. Fertil Steril 10:539, 1959.
83. Riva HL, Lawasaki DM, Messinger AJ: Further experience with norethynodrel in treatment of endometriosis. Obstet Gynecol 16:111, 1962.
84. Kistner RW: Current status of hormonal treatment of endometriosis. Clin Obstet Gynecol 9:271, 1966.
85. Kourides IA, Kistner RW: Three new synthetic progestins in the treatment of endometriosis. Obstet Gynecol 31:821, 1968.
86. Andrews WE, Larsen GD: Endometriosis: treatment with hormonal pseudopregnancy and/or operation. Am J Obstet Gynecol 118:643, 1974.
87. Karnaky KJ: The use of stilbestrol for endometriosis - preliminary report. Southern Med J 41:1109, 1948.
88. Karnaky KJ: Endometriosis JAMA 157:267, 1955.
89. Gunning JE, Moyer DL: The effect of medroxyprogesterone acetate on endometriosis in the human female. Fertil Steril 18:759, 1967.
90. Fahraeus L, Sydsjo A, Wallentin L: Lipoprotein changes durng treatment of pelvic endometriosis with medroxyprogesterone acetate. Fertil Steril 45:503, 1986.
91. Moghissi KS, Boyce CR: Management of endometriosis with oral medroxyprogesterone acetate. Obstet Gynecol 47:265, 1975.

92. Luciano AA, Turksoy RN, Carleo J: Evaluation of oral medroxyprogesterone acetate in the treatment of endometriosis. Obstet Gynecol 72:323, 1988.
93. Haney AF, Weinberg JB: Reduction of the intraperitoneal inflammation associated with endometriosis by treatment with medroxyprogesterone acetate. Am J Obstet Gynecol 159:450, 1988.
94. Cedars MI, Lu JKH, Meldrum DR, Judd JL: Treatment of endometriosis with a long acting gonadotropin-releasing hormone agonist plus medroxyprogesterone acetate. 75:641, 1990.
95. Telimaa S, Penttila I, Puolakka J, Ronnberg L, Kauppila A: Circulating lipid and lipoproteon concentrations during danazol and high-dose medroxyprotgesterone acetate therapy of endometriosis. Fertil Steril 52:31, 1989.
96. Noble AD, Letchworth AT: Treatment of endometriosis: a study of medical management. Br J of Obstet Gynecol 87:726, 1980.
97. Greenblatt RB, Tzingounis V: Danazol treatment of endometriosis: long-term follow-up. Fertil Steril 32:518, 1979.
98. Dmowski WP, Kapetanakis E, Scommegna A: Variable effects of danazol on endometriosis at 4 low-dose levels. Obstet Gynecol 59:408, 1982.
99. Moore EE, Harger JH, Rock JA, Archer DF: Management of pelvic endometriosis with low-dose danazol. Fertil Steril 36:15, 1981.
100. Barbieri RL, Evans S, Kistner RW: Danazol in the treatment of endometriosis: analysis of 100 cases with a 4-year follow-up. Fertil Steril 37:737, 1982.
101. Puleo JG, Hammond CB: Conservative treatment of endometriosis externa: the effects of danazol therapy. Fertil Steril 40:164, 1983.
102. Fedele L, Arcaina L, Bianchi S, Baglioni A, Vercellini P: Comparison of cyproterone acetate and danazol in the treatment of pelvic pain associated with endometriosis. Obstet Gynecol 73:1000, 1989.
103. Schlaff WD, Dugoff L, Damewood MD, Rock JA: Megestrol acetate for treatment of endometriosis. Obstet Gynecol 75:646, 1990.
104. Coutinho EM: Treatment of endometriosis with gestrinone (R-2323), a synthetic antiestrogen, antiprogesterone. Am J Obstet Gynecol 144:895, 1982.

105. Venturini PL, Bertolini S, Brunenghi MCM, Daga A, Fasce V, Marcenaro A, Cimato M, DeCecco L: Endocrine, metabolic, and clinical effects of gestrinone in women with endometriosis. Fertil Steril 52:589, 1989.
106. Dlugi AM, Miller JD, Knittle J, Lupron Study Group: Lupron depot (leuprolide acetate for depot suspension) in the treatment of endometriosis: a randomized, placebo-controlled, double-blind study. Fertil Steril 54:419, 1990.
107. Henzl MR, Corson SL, Moghissi K, Buttram VC, Berquist C, Jacobson J: Administration of Nasal Nafarelin as Compared with Oral Danazol for Endometriosis: A Multicenter Double-Blind Comparative Clinical Trial. N Engl J Med 318:485, 1988.
108. Rolland R, Heijden PFM van der: Nafarelin versus danazol in the treatment of endometriosis. Am J Obstet Gynecol 162:586, 1990.
109. Riis BJ, Christiansen C, Johansen JS, Jacobson J: Is it possible to prevent bone loss in young women treated with luteinizing hormone-releasing hormone agonists? J Clinical Endocrin Metab 70:920, 1990.
110. Surrey ES, Gambone JC, Lu JKH, Judd HL: The effects of combining norethindrone with a gonado-tropin-releasing hormone agonist in the treatment of symptomatic endometriosis. Fertil Steril 53:620, 1990.
111. Black WT: Use of presacral sympathectomy in the treatment of dysmenorrhea. Am J Obstet Gynecol 89:16, 1964.
112. Malinak LR: Operative management of pelvic pain. Clin Obstet Gynecol 23:191, 1980.
113. Polan ML, DeCherney A: Presacral neurectomy for pelvic pain in infertility. 34:557, 1980.
114. Garcia CR, David SS: Pelvic endometriosis: infertility and pelvic pain. Am J Obstet Gynecol 129:740, 1977.
115. Lee RB, Stone K, Magelssen D, Belts RP, Benson WL: Presacral Neurectomy for Chronic Pelvic Pain. Obstet Gynecol 68:517, 1986.
116. Perez JJ: Laparoscopic presacral neurectomy: Results of the first 25 cases. J Reprod Med 35:625, 1990.
117. Doyle JB: Paracervical uterine denervation by transection of the cervical plexus for the relief of dysmenorrhea. Am J Obstet Gynecol 70:11, 1955.
118. Lichten EM, Bombard J: Surgical treatment of primary dysmenorrhea with laparoscopic uterine nerve ablation. J Reprod Med 32:37, 1987.

119. Nezhat C, Winer WK, Nezhat F: A comparision of the CO_2 Argon, and KTP/532 lasers in the videolaseroscopic treatment of endometriosis. Colposcopy & Gynecol Laser Surgery 4:41, 1988.
120. Keye WR, Hansen LW, Astin M, Poulson AM: Argon laser therapy of endometriosis: a review of 92 consecutive patients. Fertil Steril 47:208, 1987.
121. Fayez JA, Collazo LM: Comparison between laparotomy and operative laparoscopy in the treatment of moderate and severe stages of endometriosis. Int. J Fertil 35:272, 1990.
122. Reich H, Mc Glynn F: Treatent of ovarian endometriomas using laparoscopic surgical techniques. J Reprod Med 31:577, 1986.
123. Perry CP, Upchurch JC: Pelviscopic adnexectomy. Am J Obstet Gynecl 162:79, 1990.
124. Mage G, Canis M, Manhes H, Pouly JL, Wattiez A, Bruhat MA: Laparoscopic management of adnexal cystic masses. J Gynecol Surg 6:71, 1990.
125. Goodman MP, Johns DA, Levine RL, Reish H, Levinson CJ, Murphy AA, Silva PD, Daniell JF, Diamond MP, Cropp CS: Report of the study group: advanced operative laparoscopy (pelviscopy). J Gynecol Surg 5:353, 1989.
126. Maiman M, Seltzer V, Boyce J: Laparoscopic excision of ovarian oplasms subsequently found to be malignant. Obstet Gynecol 77:563, 1991.
127. Muse K, Wilson EA, Jawad MJ: Prolactin hyper-stimulation in response to thyrotropin-releasing hormone in patients with endometriosis. Fertil Steril 38:419, 1982.
128. Haney AF, Handwerger S, Weinberg JB: Peritoneal fluid prolactin in infertile women with endometriosis: lack of evidence of secretory activity by endometrial implants. Fertil Steril 42:935, 1984.
129. Brosens IA, Koninckz PR, Corveleyn PA: A study of plasma progesterone, oestradiol-17B, prolactin, and LH levels, and of the luteal-phase appearance of the ovaries in patients with endometriosis and infertility. Br J Obstet Gynaecol 85:246, 1978.
130. Balasch J, Vanrell JA: Mild endometriosis and luteal function. Int J Fertil 30:4, 1985.
131. Wallace AM, Lees DAR, Roberts ADG, Gray CE et al: Danazol and prolactin status in patients with endometriosis. Acta Endocrinol 107:445, 1984.

132. Cheesman KL, Ben-Nun I, Chatterton RT, Cohen MR: Relationship of luteinizing hormone, pregnanediol-3-glucuronide, and estriol-16-glucronide in urine of infertile women with endometriosis. Fertil Steril 38:542, 1982.
133. Cheesman KL, Cheesman SD, Chatterton RT, Cohen MR: Alterations in progesterone metabolism and luteal function in infertile women with endometriosis. Fertil Steril 40:590, 1983.
134. Thomas EJ, Lenton EA, Cooke ID: Follicle growth patterns and endocrinological abnormalities in infertile women with minor degrees of endometriosis. Br J Obstet Gynaecol 93:852, 1986.
136. Soules MA, Malinak LR, Bury R, Poindexter A: Endometriosis and anovulation; a coexisting problem in the infertile female. Am J Obstet Gynecol 125:412, 1976.
137. Dmowski WP, Cohen MR, Wilhelm JL: Endometriosis and ovulatory failure: Does it occur? Should ovulatory stimulating agents be used. Greenblatt (ed), Recent advances in Endometriosis. Excerpta Medica pp. 129-136, 1976.
138. Badawy SZA, Nusbaum M, Taymour E: Ovulatory dysfunction in patients with endometriosis. Diagn Gynecol Obstet 3:305, 1981.
139. Ronnberg L, Kauppila A, Rajaniemi H: Luteinizing hormone receptor disorder in endometriosis. Fertil Steril 42:64, 1984.
140. Doody MC, Gibbons WE, Buttram VC: Linear regression analysis of ultrasound follicular growth series: evidence for an abnormality of follicular growth in endometriosis patients. Fertil Steril 49:47, 1988.
141. Tummon IS, Maclin VM, Radwanska E, Binor Z, Dmowski WP: Occult ovulatory dysfunction in women with minimal endometriosis or unexplained infertility. Fertil Steril 50:716, 1988.
142. Kaplan CR, Eddy CA, Olive DL, Schenken RS: Effect of ovarian endometriosis on ovulation in rabbits. Am J Obstet Gynecol 160:40, 1989.
143. Schenken RS, Asch RD, Williams RF, Hodgen GD: Etiology of infertility in monkeys with endometriosis: luteinized unruptured follicles, luteal phase defects, pelvic adhesions, and spontaneous abortions. Fertil Steril 41:122, 1984.
144. Pittaway DE, Maxson W, Daniell J, Herbert C: Luteal phase defects in infertility patients with endometriosis. Fertil Steril 39:712, 1983.

145. Dhont M, Serreyn R, Duvivier P, Vanluchene E, Boever JD, Vanderkerckhove D: Ovulation stigma and concentration of progesterone and estradiol in peritoneal fluid: relation with fertility and endometriosis. Fertil Steril 41:872, 1984.
146. Daly DC, Soto-Albors C, Walters C, Ying Y, Riddick DH: Ultrasonographic assessment of luteinized unruptured follicle syndrome in unexplained infertility. Fertil Steril 43:62, 1985.
147. Koninckx PR, Ide P, Vandenbrouke W, Brosens IA: New aspects of the pathophysiology of endometriosis and associated infertility. J Reprod Med 24:257, 1980.
148. Liukkonen S, Koskimies AI, Tenhunen A, Ylostalo P: Diagnosis of luteinized unruptured follicle (LUF) syndrome by ultrasound. Fertil Steril 41:26, 1984.
149. Brosens IA, Konickx PR, Gorveleyn PA: A study of plasma progesterone, oestradiol-17B, prolactin and LH levels, and of the luteal phase appearance of the ovaries in patients with endometriosis and infertility. Br J Obstet Gynaecol 85:246, 1978.
150. Donnez J, Langerock S, Thomas K: Peritoneal fluid volume, 17 Beta-Estradiol and progesterone concentrations in women with endometriosis and/or luteinized unruptured follicle syndrome. Gynecol Obstet Invest 16:210, 1983.
151. van Furth R, Raeburn JA, van Zwet TI: Characteristics of human mononuclear phagocytes. Blood 54:485, 1979.
152. Haney AF, Muscato JJ, Weinberg JB: Peritoneal fluid cell populations in infertility patinets. Fertil Steril 35:696, 1981.
153. Halme J, Becker S, Hammond MG, Raj MHG, Raj S: Increased activation of pelvic macrophages in infertile women with mild endometriosis. Am J Obstet Gynecol 145:333, 1983.
154. Halme J, Becker S, Wing R: Accentuated cyclic activation of peritoneal macrophages in patients with endometriosis. Am J Obstet Gynecol 148:85, 1984.
155. Badawy SZ, Cuenca V, Marshall L, Munchback R, Rinas AC, Coble DA; Cellular components in peritoneal fluid in infertile patients with and without endometriosis. Fertil Steril 42:704, 1984.
156. Halme J, Becker S, Haskill S: Altered maturation and function of peritoneal macrophages: Possible role in pathogenesis of endometriosis. Am J Obstet Gynecol 156:783, 1987.

157. Zeller JM, Henig I, Radwanska E, Dmowski WP: Enhancement of human monocyte and peritoneal macrophage chemiluminescence activities in women with endometriosis. Am J Reprod Immuno Microbiol 13:78, 1987.
158. Schenken RS, Asch RH: Surgical induction of endometriosis in the rabbit: effects on fertility and concentrations of peritoneal fluid prostaglandins. Fertil Steril 34:581, 1980.
159. Moon YS, Leung PCS, Yuen BH, Gomel_V: Prostaglandin F in human endometriotic tissue. Am J Obstet Gynecol 141:344, 1981.
160. Drake TS, O'Brien WF, Ramwell PW, Metz SA: Peritoneal fluid thromboxane B2 and 6-keto-prostaglandin F1 in endometriosis. Am J Obstet Gynecol 140:401, 1981.
161. Drake T, O'Brien W, Grunert G and Metz S: Peritoneal fluid volume in endometriosis. Fertil Steril 34:280, 1980.
162. Badawy SZA, Marshall L, Gabal AA, Nusbaum ML: The concentration of 13,14-dihydro-15-keto prostaglandin F2 and prostaglandin E2 in peritoneal fluid of infertile patients with and without endometriosis. Fertil Steril 38:166. 1982.
163. Dawood MY, Khan-Dawood FS, Wilson L: Peritoneal fluid prostaglandins and prostanoids in women with endometriosis, chronic pelvic inflammatory disease, and pelvic pain. Am J Obstet Gynecol 148:391, 1984.
164. Eisermann J, Gast MJ, Pineda J, Odem RR, Collins JL: Tumor necrosis factor in peritoneal fluid of women undergoing laparoscopic surgery. Fertil Steril 50:573, 1988.
165. Hill JA, Faris HMP, Schiff I, Anderson DJ: Characterization of leykocyte subpopulations in the peritoneal fluid of women with endometriosis. Fertil Steril 50:216, 1988.
166. Syrop CH, Halme J: A comparison of peritoneal fluid parameters of infertile patients and the subsequent occurrence of pregnancy. Fertil Steril 46:631, 1986.
167. Koninckx PR, Renair M. Brosens LA: Origin of peritoneal fluid in women: an ovarian exudation product. Br J Obstet Gynaecol 87:177, 1980.
168. Maathuis JB, VanLook PFA, Nichie EA: Changes in volume, total protein and ovarian steroid concentration of peritoneal fluid throughout the human menstrual cycle. J Endocrinol 76:123, 1978.

169. Rock JA, Dubin NH, Ghodgaonkar RB, Bergqui CA, Erozan YS, Kimball AW: Cul-de-sac fluid in women with endometriosis: fluid volume and prostanoid concentration during the proliferative phase of the cycle-days 8 to 12. Fertil Steril 37:747, 1982.
170. Rezai N. Ghodgaonkar RB, Zacur HA, Rock JA, Dubin NH: Cul-de-sac fluid in women with endometriosis: fluid volume, protein and prostanoid concentration during the periovulatory period - days 13 to 18. Fertil Steril 48:29, 1987.
171. De Leon FD, Vijayakumar R, Brown M, Rao CV, Yussman MA, Schultz G: Peritoneal fluid volume, estrogen, progesterone, prostaglandin, and epidermal growth factor concentrations in patients with and without endometriosis. Obstet Gynecol 68:189, 1986.
172. Kauma S, Clark MR, White C, Halme J: Production of fibronectin by peritoneal macrophages and concentration of fibronectin in peritoneal fluid from patients with or without endometriosis. Obstet Gynecol 72:13, 1988.
173. Joshi SG, Zamah NM, Raikar RS, Buttram VC, Henriques ES, Gordon M: Serum and peritoneal fluid proteins in women with and without endometriosis. Fertil Steril 46:1077, 1986.
174. Muscato JJ, Haney AF, Weinberg JB: Sperm phagocytosis by human peritoneal macrophages: A possible cause of infertility in endometriosis. Am J Obstet Gynecol 144:503, 1982.
175. Chacho KJ, Stronkowski Chaco M, Andresen PJ, Scommegna A: Peritoneal fluid in patients with and without endometriosis: prostanoids and macro-phages and their effect on the spermatozoa penetra-tion assay. Am J Obstet Gynecol 154:1290, 1986.
176. Stone SC, Himsl K: Peritoneal recovery of motile and nonmotile sperm in the presence of endometriosis. Fertil Steril 46:338, 1986.
177. Burke RK: Effect of peritoneal washings from women with endometriosis on sperm velocity. J Reprod Med 32:743, 1987.
178. Sueldo CE, Lambert H, Steinleitner A, Rathwick G, Swanson J: The effect of peritoneal fluid from patients with endometriosis on murine sperm-oocyte interaction. Fertil Steril 48:697, 1987.

179. Leach RE, Arneson BW, Ball SD, Ory SJ: Absence of antisperm antibodies and factors influencing sperm motility in the cul-de-sac fluid of women with endometriosis. Fertil Steril 53:351, 1990.
180. Steinleitner A, Lambert H, Kazansky C, Danks P: Peritoneal fluid from endometriosis patients affects reproductive outcome in an in vivo model. Fertil Steril 53:926, 1990.
181. Prough SG, Aksel S, Gilmore SM, Yeoman RR: Peritoneal fluid fractions from patients with endometriosis do not promote two-cell mouse embryo growth. Fertil Steril 54:927, 1990.
182. Sueldo CE, Kelly E, Montoro L, Subias E, Baccaro M, Swanson JA, Steinleitner A, Lambert H: Effect of interleukin-1 on gamete interaction and mouse embryo development. J Reprod Med 35:868, 1990.
183. Steinleitner A, Lambert H, Lauredo I: Heterologous transplantation of activated murine peritoneal macrophages inhibits gamete interaction in vivo: a paradigm for endometriosis-associated subfertility. Fertil Steril 54:725, 1990.
184. Morcos RN, Gibbons WE, Findley WE: Effect of peritoneal fluid on in vitro cleavage of 2-cell mouse embryos: possible role in infertility associated with endometriosis. Fertil Steril 44:678, 1985.
185. Damewood MD, Hesla JS, Schlaff WD, Hubbard M, Gearhart JD, Rock JA: Effect of serum from patients with minimal to mild endometriosis on mouse embryo develoment in vitro. Fertil Steril 54:917, 1990.
186. Suginami H, Yano K, Watanabe K, Matsuura S: A factor inhibiting ovum capture by the oviductal fimbriae present in endometriosis peritoneal fluid. 46:1140, 1986.
187. Suginami H, Yano K: An ovum capture inhibitor (OCI) in endometriosis peritoneal fluid: an OCI-related membrane reponsible for fimbrial failure of ovum capture. Fertil Steril 50:648, 1988.
188. Weed JC, Arquembourg PC: Endometriosis: can it produce an autoimmune response resulting in infertility? Clin Obstet Gynecol 23:885, 1980.
189. Bartosik D, Viscarello RR, Danjanoo I: Endometriosis as an autoimmune disease. Fertil Steril 41:21S, 1984.
190. Rebello R, Green FHY, Fox H: A study of the secretory immune system of the female genital tract. Br J Obstet Gynaecol 82:812, 1975.

191. Kelly JK, Fox H: The local immunological defense system of the human endometrium. J Reprod Immunol 1:39, 1979.
192. Mathur S, Peress MR, Williamson HO, et al: Autoimmunity to endometrium and ovary in endometriosis. Clin Exp Immunol 50:259, 1982.
193. Saifuddin A, Buckley CH, Fox H: Immunoglobulin content of the endometrium in women with endometriosis. Int J Gynecol Pathol 2:255, 1983.
194. Meek SC, Hodge DD, Musich JR: Autoimmunity in infertile patients with endometriosis. Am J Obstet Gynecol 158:1365, 1988.
195. Badawy SZ, Cuenca V, Stitzel A, Jacobs RDB, Tomar RH: Autoimmune phenomena in infertile patients with endometriosis. Obstet Gynecol 63:271, 1984.
196. Steele RW, Dmowski WP, Marmer DJ: Immunologic aspects of human endometriosis. Am J Reprod Immunol 6:33, 1984.
197. Wild RA, Shivers CA: Antiendometrial antibodies in patients with endometriosis. Am J Reprod Immunol Microbiol 8:84, 1985.
198. Kreiner D, Fromowitz FB, Richardson DA, Kenigsberg D: Endometrial immunofluorescence associated with endometriosis and pelvic inflammatory disease. Fertil Steril 46:243, 1986.
199. Mathur S, Chihal HJ, Homm RJ, Garzza DE, Rust PF, Williamson HO: Endometrial antigens involved in the autoimmunity of endometriosis. Fertil Steril 50:860, 1988.
200. Kennedy SH, Starkey PM, Sargent IL, Hicks BR, Barlow DH: Antiendometrial antibodies in endometriosis measured by enzyme-linked immunosorbent assay before and after treatment with danazol and nafarelin. Obstet Gynecol 75:914, 1990.
201. El-Roeiy A, Dmowski WP, Gleicher N, Radwanska E, Harlow L, Binor Z, Tommon I, Rawlins R: Danazol but not gonadotropin-releasing hormone agonists suppresses autoantibodies in endometriosis. Fertil Steril 50:864, 1988.
202. Badawy SZ, Cuenca V, Freliech H, Stefanu C: Endometrial antibodies in serum and peritoneal fluid of infertile patients with and without endometriosis. Fertil Steril 53:930, 1990.

203. Kennedy SH, Nunn B, Cederholm-Williams SA, Barlow DH: Cardiolipin antibody levels in endometriosis and systemic lupus erythematosus. Fertil Steril 52:1061, 1989.
204. Gleicher N. El-Roeiy A, Confino E, Friberg J: Is endometriosis an autoimmune disease? Obstet Gynecol 70:115, 1987.
205. Wilcox AJ, Weinberg CR, O'Connor JF, et al: Incidence of early loss of pregnancy. N Engl J Med 319:159, 1988.
206. Miller JF, Williamson E, Glue J, et al: Fetal loss after implantation: A prospective study. Lancet 2:554, 1980.
207. Edmonds DK, Lindsky KS, Miller JF, et al: Early embryonic mortality in women. Fertil Steril 38:447, 1982.
208. Grifo JA, Seifer DB: Chromosomal causes of pregnancy wastage. Infertility and Reproductive Medicine, Clinics of North America, Friedman AJ (Guest Editor), Recurrent Pregnancy Loss. WB Saunders Co., pps. 19-35, 1991.
209. Hornstein MD: Endometriosis and spontaneous abortion. Infertility and Reproductive Medicine, Clinics of North America, Recurrent Pregnancy Loss, Friedman AJ, (guest editor). W.B. Saunders Company, pps. 175-185, 1991.
210. Warburton D, Fraser FC: Spontaneous abortion risks in man: Data from reproductive histories collected in a medical genetics unit. Am J Hum Genet 16:1, 1964.
211. Shapiro S, Levine HS, Abramowicz M: Factors associated with early and late fetal loss. Adv Plann Parenthood 6:45, 1971.
212. Naylor AF, Warburton D: Sequential analysis of spontaneous abortion. II: Collaborative study data shows that gravidity determines a very substantial rise in risk. Fertil Steril 31:282, 1979.
213. Royal College of General Practitioners' Oral Contraceptive Study: The outcome of pregnancy in former oral contraceptive users. Br J Obstet Gynaecol 83:608, 1976.
214. Jansen RPS: Spontaneous abortion incidence in the treatment of infertility. Am J Obstet Gynecol 143:451, 1982.
215. Reed TE, Kelly EL: The completed reproductive performances of 161 couples selected before marriage and classified by ABO blood group. Ann Hum Genet 22:165, 1958.

216. Haydon GB: A study of 569 cases of endometriosis. Obstet Gynecol 43:704, 1942.
217. Malinak LR, Wheeler JM: Association of endometriosis with spontaneous abortion, prognosis for pregnancy, and risk for recurrence. Seminars in Reprod Endocrin 3:4, 1985.
218. Groll M: Endometriosis and spontaneous abortion. Fertil Steril 41:933, 1984.
219. Metzger DA, Olive DL, Stohs GF, Franklin RR: Association of endometriosis and spontaneous abortion: effect of control group selection. Fertil Steril 45:18, 1986.
220. FitzSimmons J, Stahl R, Gocial B, Shapiro SS: Spontaneous abortion and endometriosis. Fertil Steril 47:696, 1987.
221. Pittaway DE, Vernon C, Fayez JA: Spontaneous abortions in women with endometriosis. Fertil Steril 50:711, 1988.
222. Hahn DW, Carraher RP, Foldesy RG, McGuire JL: Experimental evidence for failure to implant as a mechanism of infertility associated with endometriosis. Am J Obstet Gynecol 155:1109, 1986.
223. Rock JA, Guzick DS, Sengos C, Schweditsch M, Sapp KC, Jones HW: The conservative surgical treatment of endometriosis: evaluation of pregnancy success with respect to the extent of disease as categorized using contemporary classification systems. Fertil Steril 35:131, 1981.
224. Naples JD, Batt RE, Sadigh H: Spontaneous abortion rate in patients with endometriosis. Obstet Gynecol 57:509, 1981.
225. Olive DL, Franklin RR, Gratkins LV: The association between endometriosis and spontaneous abortion. A Retrospective Clinical Study. J Reprod Med 27:333, 1982.
226. Schenken RS, Malinak LR: Conservative surgery versus expectant management for the infertile patient with mild endometriosis. Fertil Steril 37:183, 1982.
227. Seibel MM Berger MJ, Weinstein FG, Taymor ML: The effectiveness of danazol on subsequent fertility in minimal endometriosis. Fertil Steril 38:534, 1982.
228. Bayer SR, Seibel MM, Saffan DS, Berger MJ, Taymor ML: Efficacy of danazol treatment for minimal endometriosis in infertile women. J Reprod Med 33:179, 1988.

229. Portuondo JA, Echanojauregui AD, Herran C, Alijarte I: Early conception in patients with untreated mild endmetriosis. Fertil Steril 39:22, 1983.
230. Jansen RPS: Minimal endometriosis and reduced fecundability: prospective evidence from an artificial insemination by donor program. Fertil Steril 46:141, 1986.
231. Rodriguez-Escudero FJ, Neyro JL, Corcostegui B, Benita JA: Does minimal endometirosis reduce fecundity? Fertil Steril 50:522, 1988.
232. Kable WT, Yussman MA: Fertility after conservative treatment of endometriosis. J Reprod Med 30:857, 1985.
233. Olive DL, Stohs GF, Metzger DA, Franklin RR: Expectant management and hydrotubations in the treatment of endometriosis-associated infertility. Fertil Steril 44:35, 1985.
234. Hull ME, Moghissi KS, Magyar DF, Hayes MF: Comparison of different treatment modalities of endometriosis in infertile women. Fertil Steril 47:40, 1987.
235. Paulson JD, Asmar P, Saffan DS: Mild and moderate endometriosis. Comparison of treatment modalities for infertile couples. J Reprod Med 36:151, 1991.
236. Corson SL, Batzer FR, Gocial DC, Eisenberg E, Huppert LC, Maislin G: Surgical treatment of endometriosis at the time of gamete intrafallopian transfer. J Reprod Med 36:274, 1991.
237. Dmowski WP: Endocrine properties and clinical application of danazol. Fertil Steril 31:237, 1979.
238. Davison C, Banks W, Fritz A: The absorption, distribution and metabolic fate of danazol in rats, monkeys, and human volunteers. Arch Int Pharmacol Ther 221:294, 1976.
239. Barbieri RL: Danazol: Molecular, Endocrine, and Clinical Pharmacology. Current Concepts in Endometriosis. Proceedings of the Second International Syposium on Endometriosis held in Houston, Texas, May 1-3, 1989, Chadha DR, Buttram VC (eds), Alan R. Liss, Inc., New York, pps. 241-252, 1990.
240. Nilsson B, Sodergard R, Damber MG, Schoultz Bv: Danazol and gestagen displacement of testosterone and influence on sex-hormone-binding globulin capacity. Fertil Steril 38:48, 1982.
241. Nilsson B, Sodergard R, Damber MG, Damber JE, Schoultz Bv: Free testosterone levels during danazol therapy. Fertil Steril 39:505, 1983.

242. Carlstrom K, Doberl A, Rannevik G: Peripheral androgen levels in danazol-treated premenopausal women. Fertil Steril 39:499, 1983.
243. Steingold KA, Lu JKH, Judd HL, Meldrum DR: Danazol inhibits steroidogenesis by the human ovary in vivo. Fertil Steril 45:649, 1986.
244. Tsang BK, Henderson KM, Armstrong DT: Effect of danazol on estradiol-17B and progesterone secretion by porcine ovarian cells in vitro. Am J Obstet Gynecol 133:256, 1979.
245. Olsson JH, Hillensjo T, Nilsson L: Inhibitory effects of danazol on steroidogenesis in cultured human granulosa cells. Fertil Steril 46:237, 1986.
246. Asch RH, Fernandez EO, Siler-Khodr TM, Bartke A, Pauerstein CJ: Mechanism of induction of luteal phase defects by danazol. Am J Obstet Gynecol 136:932, 1980.
247. Henderson KM, Tsang BK: Danazol suppresses luteal function in vitro and in vivo. Fertil Steril 33:550, 1980.
248. Rabe T, Kiesel L, Runnebaum B: Inhibition of human placental progesterone synthesis by danazol in vitro. Fertil Steril 40:330, 1983.
249. Stillman RJ, Fencl MD, Schiff I, Barbieri RL, Tulchinsky D: Inhibition of adrenal steroidogenesis by danazol in vivo. Fertil Steril 33:401, 1980.
250. Holt JP, Keller D: Danazol treatment increases serum enzyme levels. Fertil Steril 41:70, 1984.
251. Wynn V: Metabolic effects of danazol. J Int Med Res (Suppl) 5:25, 1977.
252. Pearson K, Zimmerman HJ: Danazol and liver damage. Lancet 2:645, 1980.
253. Spooner JB: Classification of side-effects to danazol therapy. J Int Med Res (Suppl 3) 5:15, 1977.
254. Allen JK, Fraser IS: Cholesterol, high density lipoprotein and danazol. J Clin ENdocrinol Metab 53:149, 1981.
255. Luciano AA, Hauser KS, Chapler FK, Davis WA, Wallace RB: Effects of danazol on plasma lipid and lipoprotein levels in healthy women and in women with endometriosis. Am J Obstet Gynecol 145:422, 1983.
256. Fahraeus L, Larson-Cohn U, Ljungberg S, Wallentin L: Profound alterations of the lipoprotein metabolism during danazol treatment in premenopausal women. Fertil Steril 42:52, 1984.
257. Barbieri RL, Ryan KJ: Danazol: Endocrine

pharmacology and therapeutic applications. Am J Obstet Gynecol 141:453, 1981.
258. Bohnet HG, Hanker JP, Schweppe KW, Schneider HPG: Changes of prolactin secretion following long-term danazol application. Fertil Steril 36:725, 1981.
259. Fraser IS, Markham R, McIlveen J, Robinson M: Dynamic tests of hypothalamic and pituitary function in women treated with danazol. Fertil Steril 37:484, 1982.
260. Luciano AA, Hauser KS, Chapler FK, Sherman BM: Danazol: Endocrine consequences in healthy women. Am J Obstet Gynecol 141:723, 1981.
261. Braun P, Wildt L, Leyendecker G: The effect of danazol on gonadotropin secretion during the follicular phase of the menstrual cycle. Fertil Steril 40:37, 1983.
262. Bevan JR, Dowsett M, Jeffcoate SL: Endocrine effects of danazol in the treatment of endometriosis. Br J Obstet Gynecol 91:160, 1984.
263. Dmowski WP, Headley S, Radwanska E: Effects of danazol on pulsatile gonadotropin patterns and on serum estradiol levels in normally cycling women. Fertil Steril 39:49, 1983.
264. Hill JA, Barbieri RL, Anderson DJ: Immunosuppressive effects of danazol in vitro. Fertil Steril 48:414, 1987.
265. Mori H, Nakagawa M, Itoh N, Wada K, Tamaya T: Danzol suppresses the production of Interleukin-1B and tumor necrosis factor by human monocytes. Am J Reprod Immunol 24:45, 1990.
266. Schreiber AD, Chien P, Tomaski A, Cines DB: Effect of danazol in immune thrombocytopenic purpura. N Engl J Med 316:503, 1987.
267. Henzl MR, Kwei L: Efficacy and safety of nafarelin in the treatment of endometriosis. Am J Obstet Gynecol 162:570, 1990.
268. Goulbourne IA, Macleod DAD: An interaction between danazol and warfarin. Br J Obstet Gynecol 88:950, 1981.
269. Mercaitis PA, Peaper RE, Schwartz PA: Effect of danazol on vocal pitch: a case study. Obstet Gynecol 65:131, 1985.
270. Enyeart JJ, Price WA: Bilateral sensorineural hearing loss from danazol therapy. A case report. J Reprod Med 29:351, 1984.
271. Sikka A, Kemmann E, Vrablik RM, Grossman L: Carpal tunnel syndrome associated with danazol therapy. Am J Obstet Gynecol 147:102, 1983.

272. Duck SC, Katayama KP: Danazol may cause female pseudohermaphroditism. Fertil Steril 35:230, 1981.
273. Peress MR, Kreutner AK, Mathur RS, Williamson HO: Female pseudohermaphroditism with somatic chromosomal anomaly in association with utero exposure to danazol. Am J Obstet Gynecol 142:708, 1982.
274. Rosa FW: Virilization of the female fetus with maternal danazol exposure. Am J Obstet Gynecol 149:99, 1984.
275. Shaw RW, Farquhar JW: Female pseudohermaphroditism associated with danazol exposure in utero. Case report. Br J Obstet Gynecol 91:386, 1984.
276. Kingsbury AC: Danazol and fetal masculinization: a warning. Med J Aust 143:410, 1985.
277. Dmowski WP, Cohen MR: Antigonadotropin (danazol) in the treatment of endometriosis. Am J Obstet Gynecol 130:41, 1978.
278. Biberoglu KO, Behrman SJ: Dosage aspects of danazol therapy in endometriosis: Short-term and long-term effectiveness. Am J Obstet Gynecol 139:645, 1981.
279. Butler L, Wilson E, Belisle S, Gibson M, Albrecht B, Schiff I, Stillman R: Collaborative study of pregnancy rates following danazol therapy of stage I endometriosis. Fertil Steril 41:373, 1984.
280. Fedele L, Bianchi S, Arcaini L, Vercellini P, Candiani GB: Buserelin versus danazol in the treatment of endometriosis-associated infertility. Am J Obstet Gynecol 161:871, 1989.
281. Buttram VC: Conservative surgery for endometriosis in the infertile female: a study of 206 patients with implications for both medical and surgical therapy. Fertil Steril 31:117, 1979.
282. Buttram VC, Belue JB, Reiter R: Interim report of a study of danazol for the treatment of endometriosis. Fertil Steril 37:478, 1982.
283. Buttram VC, Reiter RC, Ward S: Treatment of endometriosis with danazol: report of a 6-year prospective study. Fertil Steril 43:353, 1985.
284. Wheeler JM, Malinak LR: Postoperative danazol therapy in infertility patients with severe endometriosis. Fertil Steril 36:460, 1981.
285. Guzick DS, Rock JA: A comparion of danazol and conservative surgery for the treatment of infertility due to mild or moderate endometriosis. Fertil Steril 40:580, 1983.

286. Donnez J, Nisolle-Pochet M, Casana-Roux F: Endometriosis-associated infertility: Evaluation of preoperative use of danazol, gestrinone, and buserelin. Int J Fert 35:297, 1990.
287. Coy DH, Schally AV: Gonadotrophin releasing hormone analogues. Ann Clin Res 10:139, 1978.
288. Stewart JM: Pharmacology of LH-RH ana analogs, in Zatuchni GI, Shelton JD, Sciarra JJ (eds): LHRH Peptides as Female and Male Contraceptives. Philadelphia, Harper & Row, p. 3, 1981.
289. Knobil E: The neuroendocrine control of the menstrual cycle. Recent Prog Horm Res 36:53, 1980.
290. Rabin D, McNeil LW: Pituitary and gonadal desensitization after continuous luteinizing hormone releasing-hormone infusion in normal females. J Clin Endocrinol Metab 51:873, 1980.
291. Friedman AJ, Harrison-Atlas D, Barbieri RL, Benacerraf B, Gleason R, Schiff I: A randomized, placebo-controlled, double-blind study evaluating the efficacy of leuprolide acetate depot in the treatment of uterine leiomyomata. Fertil Steril 51:251, 1989.
292. Friedman AJ, Barbieri RL, Benacerraf BR, Schiff I: et al: Treatment of leiomyomata with intranasal or subcutaneous leuprolide, a gonadotropin-releasing hormone agonist. Fertil Steril 48:560, 1987.
293. Matta WH, Shaw RW, Hesp R, Katz D: Hypogonadism induced by luteinizing hormone releasing hormone agonist analogues: Effects on bone density in premenopausal women. Br Med J 294:1523, 1987.
294. Tummon IA, Ali A, Pepping ME, Radwanska E, Binor Z, Dmowski WP: Bone mineral density in women with endometriosis before and during ovarian suppression with gonadotropin-releasing hormone agonist or danazol. Fertil Steril 49:792, 1988.
295. Cann CE: Reversible bone loss is produced by the GnRH agonist nafarelin, in Cohn DV, Martin JJ, Jeunier JJ (eds): Calcium Regulation and Bone Metabolism. Basic and Clinical Aspects. Amsterdam, Elsevier Science Publishers, Vol. 9, p. 123, 1987.
296. Johansen JS, Riis BJ, Hassager C, Moen M, Jacobson J, Christiansen C: The effect of a gonadotropin-releasing hormone agonist analog (nafarelin) on bone metabolism. J Clin Endocrinol Metab 67:701, 1988.
297. Matta WHM, Shaw RW, Hesp R, Evans R: Reversible

trabecular bone density following induced hypo-oestrogenism with the GnRH analogue buserelin in premenopausal women. Clin Endocrinol 29:45, 1988.

298. Dawood MY, Lewis V, Ramos J: Cortical and trabecular bone mineral content in women with endometriosis: Effect of gonadotropin releasing hormone agonist and danazol. Fertil Steril 52:21, 1989.

299. Comite F, Delman M, Hutchinson-Williams K, DeCherney AH, Jensen P: Reduced bone mass in reproductive-aged women with endometriosis. J Clin Endocrinol Metab 69:837, 1989.

300. Lane N, Baptista J, Orwoll E: Bone mineral density of the lumbar spine in women with endometriosis. Fertil Steril 55:537, 1991.

301. Jacobson JB: Effects of nafarelin on bone density. Am J Obstet Gynecol 162:591, 1990.

302. Dodin S, Lemay A, Maheux R, Dumont M, Turcot-Lemay L: Bone mass in endometriosis patients treated with GnRH agonist implant or danazol. Obstet Gynecol 77:410, 1991.

303. Huffman JW: External endometriosis. Am J Obstet Gynecol 62:1243, 1951.

304. Ranney B: Endometriosis. III. Complete operations. Reason, sequelae, treatment. Obstet Gynecol 109:1137, 1971.

305. Gray LA: Endometriosis of the bowel: Role of bowel resection, superficial excision and oophorectomy in treatment. Ann Surg 177:580, 1973.

306. Ronnberg L, Koskimies A, Laatikainen T, Ranta T, Saastamoinen J: Efficacy of gonadotropin-releasing hormone agonist (buserelin) in the treatment of endometriosis. Acta Obstet Gynecol Scand 68:49, 1989.

307. Donnez J, Nisolle-Pochet M, Clerckx-Braun F, Sandow J, Casanas-Roux F: Administration of nasal buserelin as compared with subcutaneous buserelin implant for endometriosis. Fertil Steril 52:27, 1989.

308. Clayton RN: Gonadotropin-releasing hormone modulation of its own pituitary receptors: Evidence for biphasic regulation. Endocrinology 111:152, 1982.

309. Vickery BH: Pharmacology of LHRH antagonists, in Furr BJA, Wakeling A (eds): Pharmacology and Clinical Uses of Inhibitors of Hormone Secretion and Action. London, Bailliere Tindall, P. 385, 1987.

310. Barbieri RL, Friedman AJ (eds), Gonadotropin releasing hormone analogs. Applications in gynecology. Elsevier Science Publishing Co., Inc., New York, 1991.
311. Rock JA, Guzick DS, Sengoes C, Schweditsch M, Sappo KC, Jones HW: The conservative surgical treatment of endometriosis: evaluation of pregnancy success with respect to the extent of disease as categorized using contemporary classification systems. Fertil Steril 35:131, 1981.
312. Rantala ML, Kahanpaa KV, Koskimies AI, Widholm O: Fertility prognosis after surgical treatment of pelvic endometriosis. Acta Obstet Gynecol Scand 62:11, 1983.
313. Gordts S, Boeckx W, Brosens I: Microsurgery of endometriosis in infertile patients. Fertil Steril 42:520, 1984.
314. Olive DL, Lee KC: Analysis of sequential treatment protocols for endometriosis associated infertility. Am J Obstet Gynecol 154:613, 1986.
315. Sadigh H, Naples JD, Batt RE: Conservative surgery for endometriosis in the infertile couple. Obstet Gynecol 49:562, 1977.
316. Schenken RS, Malinak LR: Reoperation after initial treatment of endometriosis with conservative surgery. Am J Obstet Gynecol 131:416, 1978.
317. Buttram VC: Surgical treatment of endometriosis in the infertile female: a modified approach. Fertil Steril 32:635, 1979.
318. Rock JA, Guzick DS, Zacur HA, Jones HW Jr.: Accessory surgical intervention in conjunction with resection and fulguration of endometriosis. Infertility 4:193, 1981.
319. Pittaway DE: Appendectomy in the surgical treatment of endometriosis. Obstet Gynecol 61:421, 1983.
320. Chong AP, Luciano A, O'Shaughnessy AM: Laser laparoscopy versus laparotomy in the treatment of infertility patients with severe endometriosis. J Gynecol Surg 6:179, 1990.
321. Cook AS, Rock JA: The role of laparoscopy in the treatment of endometriosis. Fertil Steril 55:663, 1991.
322. Daniell JF, Kurtz BR, Gurley LD: Laser laparoscopic management of large endometriomas. Fertil Steril 55:692, 1991.
323. Candiani GB, Vercellini P, Fedele L: Laparoscopic ovarian puncture for correct staging of endometriosis.

Fertil Steril 53:994, 1990.

324. Gast MJ, Tobler R, Strickler RC, Odem R, Pineda J: Laser vaporization of endometriosis in an infertile population: the role of complicating infertility factors. Fertil Steril 49:32, 1988.

325. Murphy AA, Schlaff WD, Hassiakos D, Durmusoglu F, Damewood MD, Rock JA: Laparoscopic cautery in the treatment of endometriosis-related infertility. 55:246, 1991.

326. Eward RD: Cauterization of stages I and II endometriosis and the resulting pregnancy rate. In Endoscopy in Gynecology: the Proceedings of the Third International Congress on Gynecologic Endoscopy, Edited by JM Philips. Downey, American Association of Gynecologic Laparoscopists, 1978, p 276.

327. Sulewski JM, Curcio FD, Bronitsky C, Stenger VG: The treatment of endometriosis at laparoscopy for infertility. Am J Obstet Gynecol 138:128, 1980.

328. Seiler JC, Gidwani G, Ballard L: Laparoscopic cauterization of endometriosis for fertility: a controlled study. Fertil Steril 46:1098, 1986.

329. Nowroozi K, Chase JS, Check JH, Wu CH: The importance of laparoscopic coagulation of mild endometriosis in infertile women. Int J Fertil 32:442, 1987.

330. Kelly RW, Roberts DK: CO_2 laparoscopy. A potential alternative to danazol in the treatment of stage I and II endometriosis. J Reprod Med 28:638, 1983.

331. Feste JR: Laser laparoscopy: a new modality. J Reprod Med 30:413, 1985.

332. Martin DC: CO_2 laser laparoscopy for endometriosis associated with infertility. J Reprod Med 31:1089, 1986.

333. Davis GD: Management of endometriosis and its associated adhesions with the CO_2 laser laparoscope. Obstet Gynecol 68:422, 1986.

334. Donnez J: CO_2 laser laparoscopy in infertile women with endometriosis and women with adnexal adhesions. Fertil Steril 48:390, 1987.

335. Sutton C, Hill D: Laser laparoscopy in the treatment of endometriosis. A 5-year study. Br J Obstet Gynaecol 97:181, 1990.

336. Fayez JA, Collazo LM, Vernon C: Comparison of different modalities of treatent for minimal and mild endometriosis. Am J Obstet Gynecol 159:927, 1988.

337. Nezhat C, Crowgey S, Nezhat F: Videolaseroscopy for the treatment of endometriosis associated with infertility. Fertil Steril 51:237, 1989.
338. Olive DL, Martin DC: Treatment of endometriosis-associated infertility with CO_2 laser laparoscopy: the use of one-and two-parameter expotential models. Fertil Steril 48:18, 1987.
339. Keye WR, Matson GA, Dixon J: The use of the argon laser in the treatment of experimental endometriosis. Fertil Steril 39:26, 1983.
340. Badawy SZA, Choe JK, Cohn G, Refaie A, Stefanu C, Cuenca V: Argon laser laparoscopy for treatment of pelvic endometriosis associated with infertility and pelvic pain. J Gynecol Surg 7:27, 1991.
341. Lomano JM: Photcoagulation of early pelvic endometriosis with the Nd:YAG laser through the laparoscope. 30:77, 1985.
342. Corson SL, Unger M, Kwa D, Batzer FR, Gocial B: Laparoscopic laser treatment of endometriosis with the Nd:YAG sapphire probe. Am J Obstet Gynecol 160:718, 1989.
343. Corson SL, Woodland M, Frishman G, Batzer FR, Gocial B, Maislin G: Treatment of endometriosis with a Nd:YAG tissue-contact probe via laparoscopy. Int J Fertil 34:284, 1989.
344. Corson SL: Use of the YAG laser in laparoscopic gynecologic procedures. Obstet Gynecol Clin of N. Am 18:619-636, 1991.
345. Kojima E, Yanagibori A, Yuda K, Hirakawa S: Nd:YAG laser endoscopy. J Reprod Med 33:907, 1988.
346. Shirk GJ: Use of the Nd:YAG laser for the treatment of endometriosis. Am J Obstet Gynecol 160:1344, 1989.
347. Dodson WC, Whitesides DB, Hughes CL, Easley HA, Haney AF: Superovulation with intrauterine insemination in the treatment of infertility: a possible alternative to gamete intrafallopian transfer and in vitro fertilization. Fertil Steril 48:441, 1987.
348. Corson SL, Batzer FR, Gocial B, Maislin G: Intrauterine insemination and ovulation stimulation as treatment of infertility. J Reprod Med 34:397, 1989.
349. Deaton JL, Gibson M, Blackmer KM, Nakajima ST, Badger GJ, Brumsted JR: A randomized, controlled trial of clomiphene citrate and intrauterine insemination in

couples with unexplained infertility or surgically corrected endometriosis. Fertil Steril 54:1083, 1990.

350. Mahadevan MM, Trounson AO, Leeton JF: The relationship of tubal blockage, infertility of unknown cause, suspected male infertility, and endometriosis to success of in vitro fertilization and embryo transfer. Fertil Steril 40:755, 1983.

351. Matson PL, Yovich JL: The treatment of infertility associated with endometriosis by in vitro fertilization. Fertil Steril 46:432, 1986.

352. Chillik CF, Acosta AA, Garcia JE, Perera S, Van Uem JFHM, Rosenwaks Z, Jones HW: The role of in vitro fertilization in infertile patients with endometriosis. Fertil Steril 44:56, 1985.

353. Oehninger S, Acosta AA, Kreiner D, Muasher SJ, Jones HW Jr, Rosenwaks Z: In vitro fertilization and embryo transfer (IVF:ET): an established and successful therapy for endometriosis. J In Vitro Fert Embryo Trans 5:249, 1988.

354. Oehninger S, Rosenwaks Z: In vitro fertilization and embryo transfer: an established and successful therapy for endometriosis. Progress in Clinical and Biological Research, Vol. 323, Current Concepts in Endometriosis. Chadha DR, Buttram VC (eds). Alan R. Liss, Inc., pps. 319-335, 1990.

355. Hulme VA, van der Merwe JP, Kruger TF: Gamete intrafallopian transfer as treatment for infertility associated with endometriosis. Fertil Steril 53:1095, 1990.

356. Gindoff PR, Hall JL, Nelson LM, Stillman RJ: Efficacy of assisted reproductive technology during diagnostic and operative infertility laparoscopy. Obstet Gynecol 75:299, 1990.

357. Remorgida V, Anserini P, Croce S, Costa M, Ferraiolo A, Capitanio GL: Comparison of different ovarian stimulation protocols for gamete intrafallopian transfer in patients with minimal and mild endometriosis. Fertil Steril 53:1060, 1990.

358. Batzofin J, Tran C, Tan T, Blank W, Norbryhn G, Serafini P: Laser laparoscopy as an adjunct to assisted reproductive treatments in women with pelvic adhesions and endometriosis. J Gynecol Surg 5:273, 1989.

359. Damewood MD, Rock JA: Treatment independent

pregnancy with operative laparoscopy for endometriosis in an in vitro fertilization program. Fertil Steril 50:463, 1988.

360. Punnonen R, Klemi P, Nikkanen V: Recurrent endometriosis. Gynecol Obstet Invest 11:307, 1980.
361. Candiani GB, Fedele L, Vercellini P, Bianchi S, Di Nola G: Repetitive conservative surgery for recurrence of endometriosis. Obstet Gynecol 77:421, 1991.
362. Wheeler JM, Malinak LR: Recurrent endometriosis: Incidence, management, and prognosis. Am J Obstet Gynecol 146:247, 1983.